BATTLE COURAGE

Channeling My Inner Warrior Princess
to Kick Cancer's Ass

Kaye Henrickson

Orange Hat Publishing
www.orangehatpublishing.com - Waukesha, WI

For information, please contact:

Orange Hat Publishing
www.orangehatpublishing.com
603 N Grand Ave, Waukesha, WI 53186

Edited by Christine Woods
Cover design by Therese Joanis
Cover photo credit: Heidi Baken of HB Photography

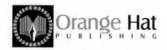

www.orangehatpublishing.com

Dedication

Name Disclaimer: You are going to see names in place of my given name, Kaye. During our first meeting, my husband, Dave, and I hilariously got each other's names wrong. I thought he was "Henri," and he thought I was "Kayla." It stuck. It's still funny. Also, my close family members call me "Kacee." I was supposed to be a boy, or so I heard through family stories. So, Kacee, it is. Not as funny as the Kayla story, but it's still close to my heart.

To Henri (Dave),

This is all you.

I'd still be balled up in the fetal position, toasting at my own pity party and sobbing uncontrollably about everything from radiation burns to medication reactions to dog hair on the couch. My wings were clipped, and I crashed to the ground. You taught me how to fly without wings. You taught me how to focus on the good—the good in absolutely everything. You taught me how to laugh again. Like really belly laugh. You taught me that light shines the brightest on the darkest nights. You taught me how to love unconditionally. You taught me how to breathe again.

Love you madly,

"Kayla"

To Ashley and Jordan,

You are my soul and my spirit. I've said this since the day each of you was born. You are who I want to make the proudest because that's what you have given me. You've given me a beautiful purpose to be the best version of myself I can be. That doesn't always happen; I know that. Yet you still allow me to be your mom.

All my love,

Mom

To A.M., B.D., K.J., and K.P. (and any future grands who may bless my heartspace),

You are my light. Because of you, I have hope. Because of you, I have deeper purpose. Because of you, I have stories to share and wisdom to impart. Because of you, I am young again. Because of you, I am. You are the best pieces of me.

I will love you. Forever.

Gaga

To Shell, Trish, and Mom,

The only thing I can say is I'm sorry for the younger, more heinous version of me. You are all miracles, and it only took fifty years to figure it out. Now who's the smart one?

Love you,

Kacee

To My Sisters in Pink,

Some of us have been friends or known each other for years. Some of us have recently found our lives intersecting at this crazy and crooked crossroads. If I had to thank cancer for anything, it is the gift of you. You make me better. All of you.

Deepest love and gratitude,

Kaye

Table of Contents

Introduction

You may write me down in history
With your bitter, twisted lies,
You may trod me in the very dirt
But still, like dust, I'll rise.

Does my sassiness upset you?
Why are you beset with gloom?
'Cause I walk like I've got oil wells
Pumping in my living room.

Just like moons and like suns,
With the certainty of tides,
Just like hopes springing high,
Still I'll rise.

Did you want to see me broken?
Bowed head and lowered eyes?
Shoulders falling down like teardrops,
Weakened by my soulful cries?

Does my haughtiness offend you?
Don't you take it awful hard
'Cause I laugh like I've got gold mines
Diggin' in my own backyard.

You may shoot me with your words,
You may cut me with your eyes,
You may kill me with your hatefulness,
But still, like air, I'll rise.

Does my sexiness upset you?
Does it come as a surprise
That I dance like I've got diamonds
At the meeting of my thighs?

Out of the huts of history's shame
I rise
Up from a past that's rooted in pain
I rise
I'm a black ocean, leaping and wide,
Welling and swelling I bear in the tide.

Leaving behind nights of terror and fear
I rise
Into a daybreak that's wondrously clear
I rise
Bringing the gifts that my ancestors gave,
I am the dream and the hope of the slave.

I rise

I rise

I rise.

Dr. Maya Angelou always finds a way to impact me deeply with her words. This poem, "Still I Rise," and volumes of others like it reside on my nightstand. I received her books of poetry as a high school graduation gift what seems like a hundred years ago, but her words are timeless. Turns out, Dr. Angelou has had to prop me up a few times throughout my first half-century on Earth. Only this time, I was going to need her wisdom more than I could have ever anticipated.

Adversity isn't novel. It isn't even special. Sometimes it's the elephant in the room. Sometimes it's the mouse running around . . . maybe up your pant leg. It might be a mountain. It might be a molehill. The point is, each one of us has experienced adversity: the time we got benched during the basketball game, the time a spouse cheated or racked up all kinds of online gambling debt, the time our career took an unexpected nosedive, the time our precious family fur baby crossed over the rainbow bridge. The horrifying beauty about adversity is that it comes in all sizes—one size does not fit all. There is no "one size fits all" way to cope, either.

This book took me over fifty years to write. When you're dealt heavy bouts of life's trials time and time again, I guess you really don't think about it much; you just figure out what needs to be done to move forward. There are lulls in the craziness, and things are fantastic. Even serenely and blissfully mundane, to some extent. Then, out of nowhere, the freight train hits, and it's time to board whether you bought a ticket or not. Some rides last longer than others. Sometimes you're seated uncomfortably inside the racing steel giant, and sometimes you're hanging onto the rail for dear life, outside, in the freezing rain, going ninety miles an hour . . . and you're approaching a tunnel. A narrow one. Some rides leave scratches. Some leaves scars. Mine was a doozy!!

As I mentioned before, this is my journey. I'm uncertain if I possess any clear answers, really. Frankly, I have more questions than answers most of the time. I've learned that there are no quick fixes when you deal with cancer. Much like the mythological Amazon warriors never really "got done" with battling over territory, over vengeance, over protection of their precious homeland of Ephesus, you don't ever "get done" with cancer, either. This was a complete misconception of mine up until now. I'm 99.9 percent certain I didn't do everything "by the book," but cancer diagnoses are undeniably unique, and I guess the warrior princess in me said, "I'll do things the way I want . . . or can." I've repeated this mantra time and time again in so many different situations. Every battle is different. Every battle requires its own plan of attack and strategy. Every battle requires a strong cadre of warriors. But no matter how prepared we might think we are for battle, know that even warrior princesses can be broken into pieces.

This book is a memoir of sorts. Reflections from a ridiculously contemplative soul during a ridiculously contemplative period in my life. I ruminate way too much. This may shock those who know me best, but yes, I spend an inordinate amount of time rummaging around inside my own noodle. I want this book to be cathartic. But I hope it connects to you, dear reader, on some level as well. You picked this book up for a reason. Maybe you were curious to see what I had to say. Maybe you sought a little sensible, down-to-earth practicality in the garbage truck of tribulation in your own life. Maybe you're my family or friends, and I pleaded with you to purchase a few copies and dole them out as gifts to everyone you knew. Thank you, by the way, if you did indeed do that. As the reader, you hold the power to make your own world-text connections. Insert your own adversity—we all have it at some level—at any point in my story. My adversity just happens to be "The Big C." Take what helps and ditch the rest. And I'm not offended too easily . . . not anymore.

One request: If you find yourself feeling the itch to reach out and do something for those going through a hellhole of their own, DO IT. Find a way to support them and their loved ones. Sometimes the people who struggle the most are too preoccupied with struggling to even know how to respond to, "How can I help?" Most times we don't have a clue. We're just trying to make it to the next hour, the next day, the next phase. Cure cancer, maybe? Reverse time? Take the pain away? Those would be all sorts of awesomesauce. But since that's unrealistic, try a phone call, a text, a Facebook message, or a card. It can be soup, gift cards for a nice meal out between treatments, a pan of scotcharoos (my personal fave), or a walk just to chat in the spring sunshine. Knowing there are people out there who sincerely care is half the battle. From what I've experienced, sometimes we think we can do this on our own. Sadly, many do exactly that—they do this on their own. Don't let them. Sharing my story is my modest attempt to help. I used to be *that* person. "I'll do it myself. I'll figure it out. I'll be fine." Lie. Lie. Lie.

Early in my journey, my work family asked me what they could do for me. I didn't have a clue. Positive thoughts, maybe? Prayers, if they were the praying type? Mantras and meditation juju sent in my general direction? It all seemed pretty vague to me, but you know what that creative crew of compassion did? They gifted me a lovely blue box with my first initial displayed on the top. Inside were etched notes of positivity, some scribed on a sticky note, some elaborately decorated. Some hilariously inappropriate. Some straight from their respective books of faith. To this day, every time I open the "positive vibes" box and the unique messages shared in cards or posts, it feeds my soul and lifts my spirit. The kindness and encouragement showered on my husband, Dave, and me during our journey could not go unnoticed, so you'll see a sampling of the countless uplifting messages throughout the book. They are subtle, sincere, and moving reminders that we are never alone. Insert your challenge, make a connection, and battle on in true warrior fashion!

Thanks for picking up the book.

Chapter 1: What's With the Warrior Princess Stuff, Anyway?

{
I have learned over the years that when one's mind is made up,
this diminishes fear.
~Rosa Parks~
}

I'll admit it. During the '90s, I shamelessly binged watched *Xena: Warrior Princess*. Binge-watching in the '90s, you ask? Yes. I guess I'm an unintentional trendsetter that way. Friends can attest to the fact that I did indeed dress as Xena for Halloween one year. Long ago. When it was okay to go out in public dressed like that. I was entertained by how actress Lucy Lawless depicted a strong, albeit scantily clad, fictional and mythical Amazon warrior. That sparked my desire to learn more about the Amazons—the buxom, tall, strong goddesses who went to war. None of them would meet today's industry standard of what a beautiful, strong woman is *supposed* look like . . . or act like, for that matter. I loved that! Thank goodness some of that stereotypical perception is evolving, however slowly. They were sassy, smart, savvy, and probably pretty harsh with their words, their wisdom, and their weapons.

Dang, could they throw a spear! I identified. Not with the Xena version but with the large-framed, strong-bodied, snarky-tongued fighter. Perhaps more with Penthesilea, the Queen of the Amazons. According to everything I could find on her, she was one forceful, horse-riding, enemy-slaughtering embodiment of Amazon spirit: active, courageous, beautiful, and brave. She was also incredibly flawed. Oh boy, do I get that. Don't get me wrong. In true warrior princess fashion, I would expect anyone donning that warrior identity to do exactly what they want, the way they want. I had originally intended to entitle this book, *Warrior Princesses Don't Wear Bikinis*. Because I have amazing friends and colleagues who challenge my perception, I got thinking. These Amazon warriors did what they had to in order to get the job done, and it might have been in a bikini, or it might not have. So, my fellow warriors, choose to sport that bikini and own it if you want. Heck, go naked into battle if it works better for you . . . or don't. Just be your own warrior. Choose your own path. Do YOU.

One interesting, and incredibly ironic, factoid that popped up continuously as I researched the Amazons was a myth that they were thought to have cut off one breast in order to better fire an arrow or hurl a spear. The notion was that the actual word, "Amazon," was Greek for "one breast." It's long been disputed by historians as well as folk etymologists, but it felt a little true to me. All medical ramifications aside (e.g. bleeding to death), it struck a chord. One breast. Hmmmm . . .

Amazons defied everything. Women and men were equals, in all things, especially war. Amazons were risk takers. I was drawn to the concept of oppositional defiance before it was recognized as a "thing," and the sheer notion of using physicality as motivation to protect and defy was exceptionally pleasing to me. I'm pretty sure I was all that and then some as a developing child, adolescent, and young adult. If the sky was blue, I'd argue it was some sort of teal. I was certainly problematic as a developing child (sorry, Mom). It got me into a lot of trouble. A lot. Let's face it: I was a brat! Ask my sisters. As an adult, with an odd propensity to reflect, I have softened my edges a bit, but I sure as hell would not be wearing a bikini . . . unless I wanted to, of course. I can only imagine Amazons did pretty much what they wanted the way they wanted to do it, too. They showed little mercy for their foes, were loyal to a fault, and—this was the best part—Amazons donned some pretty gnarly tattoos. Wow! Who knew? I completely identified. I unabashedly related to them. I, too, was often "uncoachable" and headstrong. It takes a special individual with incredible insight and a knack for dredging through the murkiness of the code of oppositional defiance and nurture it into something positive. I happen to be married to one of those people. He has softened my edges while honoring my feisty spirit. Turns out, I would need that spark plug of uncompromising, spear-slinging defiance to carry me through this quagmire. I needed to defy naysayers. I needed to defy self-perceived doom. I needed to defy cancer.

I've always wanted to write a book. Any book. Some book. What book? An "I don't know" book. I knew I had content. I had stories to tell. We all do. At my age, I've certainly lived long enough to have been bullied, to have bullied, to have experienced abuse in varying magnitudes, to have made some pretty dumb mistakes—both laughable and just downright stupid. To have had unshakeable faith, to have lost my faith, to have rediscovered my faith. I've traveled, I've had some pretty empowering career opportunities, and I've suffered heart-wrenching loss. I've got a family that rivals none. I have friend circles I'd pit against anyone. So what the heck do I write about? Living half a century doesn't necessarily make you a guru of anything, really. It just makes you fifty years old or older. Writing a book is scary. What if readers don't relate? What if judgment is harsh and swift? What if it offends someone? What if it ends up collecting dust in someone's bathroom and no one reads it until it's ultimately discarded to fire up the woodstove? Those kinds of fears floated away once I made up my mind. And in true warrior princess form, I chose to stand up for what I knew and share it so I might, in some remote way, lift up someone else and encourage them to stand up too. I am only able to do this because others have lifted me up throughout my journey. Warriors never enter battle alone. Enter mindshift: What if this actually connects with someone in some small way and they find value in it? What if it reaches someone, letting him know he's not alone? What if she cries because the words—all of them—the good, the nasty, and offensive resonate and give her a voice of her own? What if it ends up mangled and highlighted and written all over in its margins? Cool.

Like a lone star glistening brightly in a black night sky, there it was. Purpose. I *wanted* to write this book. I *needed* to write this book. I did not, however, *want* to get cancer.

It seems my whole life, up until this diagnosis, I'd been fighting something. Most times, I wasn't sure what I was fighting. It just always seemed like I needed a cause to be passionate about. To fight with all my might. To defend to the core. Growing up, it was justice. It was attention. It was self-esteem. It was being that edgy square peg trying to squeeze into a perfectly round, popular, preppy hole. That did not always work out well. I wasn't popular. I wasn't from the right side of the tracks. I didn't have a nuclear family or designer clothes or the latest hair style. I knew I was different from the get-go. Being different sucks sometimes when you're young, trying to fit in, make your mark, and get the recognition you think you deserve. Our formative teen years are those years when we first experience the opportunities of choosing *bitter* or *better*. Much like most inexperienced-at-life teens, I chose a cocktail of both. It wasn't always pretty.

Next came fighting for family. Fight-to-the-death, not always effective, "mother bear" parenting and partnering. Mess with my family and well, you know the rest. I was determined to be a good mother, wife, and, when necessary, head of household. Yes, "head" of household. Luckily, I had (and still have) a fabulous husband. We have been true partners throughout our entire lives together—good, bad, or indifferent. There were times when it became necessary for me to be head of household. There were times when Dave took over the reins. Our roles fluctuated depending on the situation we faced. There were moments of unsubstantiated anger. There were moments of sheer success. There were mostly moments of learning as we went, just trying to keep one nostril above water. It's been a true tag team partnership from the start.

Throughout my thirties and forties, it was a freakish passion for fitness, and of course, in true "I don't do moderation" Kaye fashion, I went way overboard. Severely limiting nutrition choices to basically air and twigs and excessive hours of workout time became unsustainable, and frankly, quite ludicrous. So I stopped. Dieting. Exasperating workouts. Cold turkey. Going nuts about fitness wasn't my most stellar idea. It's all about balance, and now I'm really trying not to be *that* "all in or all out" person. Moderation just eludes me for some reason. Then, with children flying the nest, my attention turned to career passions of equity and access for all students and rural students and inner city students and poverty and yes, politics. I despise almost everything about politics, political correctness, "standard operating procedures," and how they tend to rear their ugly heads to divide and stifle us as opposed to unite and propel us forward. Ugh. Enough with the passion projects already. Enough with the fighting for whatever cause. It's exhausting trying to keep up. Always a *warrior*. Sometimes without a clue or without a plan, but always a *warrior*. The thing is, when I think about the whole warrior princess thing, no one I know would likely ever use a descriptor like "princess" to describe me. They would probably choke on their laughter if they heard I was a princess!

Truth is, I clearly *am* a princess. Maybe not Sleeping Beauty waiting to be kissed by my Prince Charming, but a princess, nonetheless. Think about it: I live in a beautiful castle built by my knight in shining armor. He rescued me from some pretty horrendous, fire-breathing dragons. I can blissfully wander away my days with my children and grands frolicking in the meadow, or in our case, the woods. I come and go pretty much as I please on trusty steeds made of iron and steel. I work on matters of the heart to my heart's content. I live a charmed life. Bills get paid. Beds are warm. Bellies are full. Every text, every goodbye, every day ends with, "I love you." Yep. *Princess.*

That doesn't mean princesses don't know how to fight, like a Fiona-type, Shrek princesses—some are *warriors*, too. Just by virtue of being labelled *princess* affords some type of license to do as one wishes—like not wear bikinis or plaster your body with tattoos. Unless, of course, your name is Leia, you have Cinnabons® on your head, and it's 1983 in a galaxy far, far away . . . and, you want to. My point is, life is a choice. How you navigate through all of the muck is also a choice. How you celebrate the wonder is, too. Let's be honest—there are clearly moments of triumph, moments to be proud of, and moments that quite frankly bring you to your knees, pleading for mercy. Sometimes wonder comes in actually tasting the P, the B, and the J in a PB & J again. Sometimes wonder comes in a grandchild's eyes. Sometimes wonder is waking to an ethereal, serene sunrise with limbs that no longer tingle in pain.

As I looked through an old wooden treasure box I had made probably some time during my woodworking class days in junior high (we didn't call it middle school in the good ol' days), I came across some old report cards, faded senior photos, and a host of notes handwritten on folded, progressively crusty-ing paper. I have to admit, some were painful to read. Some were clear reflections of the hilarity and drama that comprised my teenhood angst. They brought to life memories I had long suppressed. Everything bubbled and boiled to the top of my heart—how horrible I was to my sisters during my formative years, how awful I must have been to raise, how troubled I was in my teens, lying to fit in with the "cool kids," making choices that only led to self-harm just to feel loved, how my true friends and loved ones at the time tried with all their might to correct the course of my path only to be kicked in the teeth. Holy repressed memories! I harbored a lot of anger back then. Something was obviously askew during that period of my life, as it is with many of us. Let's face it—we all can look back and identify things we wish we could either erase or travel back in time to revise. But it's part of growing up and growing older. With tremendous effort and a safety net support system that rivals none, I learned to channel the anger into passion projects, transition negative into positive, and, for the most part, move forward to grow, mature, and become a better version of my spunky self. My first grade teacher nailed it, though. She framed an ancient paper report card, hand scribing a lengthy narrative around all my "exceeds" and "satisfactories" to extol my inherent "leadership" qualities:

Kaye is a natural leader. She needs to realize that others need a chance.

Kaye excels in all curricular areas; however, she tends to be bossy on the playground and during lunch.

Kaye finishes her work quite speedily and often finishes her classmates' work without giving them a chance to show what they know. She needs to realize not everyone can complete tasks as readily as she does.

This last comment was damn funny. Even at seven, I was a closer. It's interesting how, even though we mature and change as we age, the core of who we are remains intact. Even at an early age, I didn't like to see others struggle. That hasn't changed. Subsequently, I find myself doing things all by myself and doing things for others so they don't have to. Funny how cancer can shift things. For the first time in my life, I was faced with a situation I couldn't do all on my own. Humbling.

Mrs. F. nailed it. She understood me. Fast forward another forty-some odd years, and I need this seven-year-old version of myself again. This spicy seven-year-old needs to boss her way through this fight. She needs to harness that assertiveness to beat down an enemy. Keeping my first-grade teacher's observations in mind, I cling to the Amy Poehler quote, "Bossy is not a pejorative term. It means someone is passionate and engaged and ambitious." Combine the two in a bowl, mix thoroughly until blended, serve hot.

When you're thrown for a loop (and cancer is one helluva loop on the old roller coaster ride), the "deer in the headlights" reaction only works for a little while. That's what happened to me. Reviving that saucy, bossy seven-year-old who grew into a warrior was the only way I could survive. We were headed for battle, kids! This warrior princess, bikini or not, had to sharpen up the spear and spit shine the armor because it was a battle I had absolutely NO CLUE how to fight. All I knew for sure was that retreat was not an option.

This note I received from a friend cracks me up every single time I read it. It brought smiles through tears, light when it was challenging to traverse the darkness:

Tough Cookie (tuhf kook-e): *noun*
Someone with just the right mix of sweetness and strength.
One who doesn't crumble under pressure.

A fighter who's too busy kicking butt to sit down and cry, but knows it's okay to do both.

A person who doesn't always ask for support, but has lots of friends who would do anything to help.

Kaye,

I thought this was a perfect description of you! So sorry you have to deal with it! Prayers your way!

A.S.

Chapter 2: The Bitch Slap

{ *Two roads diverged in a wood, and I—I took the one less traveled by,*
and that has made all the difference.
~Robert Frost~ }

Pardon the profanity of this chapter's title, but the truth can be ugly sometimes . . . and vulgar. There's no gentle way to describe how it feels when a doctor says, "We think it's cancer." There's no grace in trying to hold back a waterfall of snot and blubbering when you hear the news. There's no grace in bawling to your husband over the phone, so wrought with sobs you physically cannot leave the hospital parking lot. There is no grace in being presented with options that can only be seen as torture . . . hopefully with survival as the end game. There are numerous individuals I know and admire who have this insane propensity for grace under fire. I'm reminded of the mythological Amazons. They were quick-witted, calm, and focused on winning the battle. They collaborated, they strategized, and they each knew their role. The moment I learned my fate, I wished I could have been more like those warriors I so admired, both mythical and real . . . but alas, it just was not part of my DNA. I was so incredibly frightened, and when I get scared, I immediately get angry. But I bet the Amazons were a little scared sometimes, too. Maybe, for both them and for me, anger turns to courage. Courage to go to battle. So guess what, cancer? This means war.

Journal Entry: January 23rd

Seventeen days ago I received my diagnosis. Almost a month ago, on the day after Christmas, I found something unusual in my breast. Today, I realized I am never going to be the same. Some days I am filled with hope and determination. Other days, fear. Breast cancer isn't the death sentence it once was, but it sure isn't for wimps—or the impatient.

For me, in times of crisis and weakness, I seek power in knowledge—facts, data, research—from reputable sources. It's amazing to me how open-hearted some people become when they hear you've been diagnosed with breast cancer. We all know a survivor or ten. Well, I did not. Not really. I knew OF women who had been diagnosed with breast cancer who now lead full lives. I did not, however, know the extent of their journey until I was thrust into it myself. Now, I needed to wrap my head around as much factual information as I could gather, not just do some innocuous Google search, only to find a flux of "fact" and rampant horror stories. Give me facts. Give me information. Give me options. Give me hope. That's the only way I'm going to ever regain power and control over my journey. I'm a control freak. Control freaks need facts.

My facts have taken what seems like an eternity to obtain. Three "suspicious" areas on the right breast led to a core needle biopsy, which led to the diagnosis of DCIS (pretty stagnant, isolated ductal cancer). Don't worry; I needed to write this all down because it really never registered in my brain until now. Then, there remained this issue of the cancer wandering into my axillary lymph nodes—but, they weren't metastatic, which I have since learned is a very, very, VERY big deal. They were just there, hanging out—how the hell did they get there?

This led to multiple MRI biopsies. We couldn't do all this work on the right side without ensuring the left side was clean. Well, it wasn't. There was something "suspicious" going on over there, too. Great. We also found another cluster of trouble under the right side, next to the chest wall. Could this be the culprit? Was this the source? Only another biopsy would tell. Super.

So . . . three weeks have passed since my initial diagnosis. I have read, and reread, as much information as my brain (and soul) could digest—and to be honest, I'm getting twitchy. I dotted all my i's and crossed all my t's at work. As we wait, I try to fill my thoughts with tasks, plans, lists—all so I can have some semblance of control and order before all hell breaks loose.

We had planned a trip to Cancun last August (2016) to celebrate Dave's retirement, his birthday, and Valentine's Day. We had saved and saved for months and months for this trip. It was happening, damn it! A roadtrip to El Paso with four cats, four potty/gas stops, a really old iTunes playlist, eight venison sandwiches, four Mountain Dews, and 5-Hour Energy® for a twenty-two hour stint? Yeah—that happened. Don't ask why; we love our kids. Tickets to Phantom of the Opera *for a girls' weekend? So happened! After all that? I was told to keep my calendar light. Yeah. Light. I didn't even know what that meant.*

This was supposed to be a pea-sized bump. This was supposed to be compassionate but stern conversations revolving around eating more kale, getting more exercise, dissolving fatty tissue, testing the thyroid, keeping those happy little hormones in check. Nope. Not the conversation I had even remotely expected. Then again, no one EXPECTS to hear, "You've got the Big C." I can't fathom anyone being mentally prepared to respond to this news properly. Is there even a proper way? If there is a proper way to handle any of this, I sure missed the memo.

Alas, according to United States breast cancer statistics from BreastCancer.org, one in eight women in the US will be diagnosed with breast cancer. One in eight. I thought about all of the circles of females in my life. No one in my close friend circles had it. Yes, a few work colleagues had been diagnosed . . . not near the one in eight. None of my female relatives had full-blown breast cancer, complete with a full menu of treatment options. I could count on one hand those in my extended female acquaintance/friend circles impacted. But I guess I won. I got to be the one in eight. I've always considered myself to be somewhat of a pioneer . . . or guinea pig. Someone always eager to try new things, be an "early adopter," test the waters of a new travel destination or an exotic culinary delight. I like to think I live a life of reckless abandon which, all things considered, turns out to be a ludicrous notion when faced with cancer. Let's try ghost peppers once. Let's travel somewhere no one speaks English. Let's navigate down a new waterway with our kayaks. Let's be stupid. Let's be adventurous. Let's ask questions later and have no regrets.

Nope. Not. This.

The memory of hearing a dear friend comment, "At least you have the good cancer," still throws me into a tailspin of "whatthehell" every time. That one was a slap. I'm relatively certain it came from a good place, from a place of confusion and compassion. At least, I hope it was. Yes, I am acutely aware that of all cancers, breast cancer tends to be the most curable and among the highest funded. What else would you expect from a bunch of women (and yes, men) with their backs—and breasts—pinned up against a wall? Of course, there's action. And funding. And cures. I know that. Because I try to understand the motivations behind people's comments, I really struggled with this one. Maybe I misread it. Was it lack of understanding? Was it a loss for words? Was it an impulsive, albeit awkward, statement that frequently follows shock? However compassionate and uplifting this statement was meant to be, I'll be honest. I found it hurtful. Answer me this: Is *any* kind of cancer the *good* kind?

How was I supposed to react? What's the normal etiquette for handling cancer with grace and composure anyway? It's so hard to know. I got cancer the year I turned fifty. Turning fifty was kind of a big deal for me, but not necessarily in a bad way. It just felt like I had arrived at a positive pinnacle in my life—that I could look forward, and I could look back. I was on a roll. I had raised kids with the man I had loved all my life. We had grown and transformed and battled to remain people *we* would want to hang out with. I did not want a big party. I wanted to welcome in the next half-century with big dreams, big goals, big ideas for the next fifty! Cancer only added to that feeling—that we are not going to be here forever. *Are you living your life the way you want it to be? What are the things you've always wanted to do or meant to do? You're still here, and you're fifty. Why the hell aren't you doing them?* It sounds like such a little thing, but I took up playing the piano and returned to my writing roots again. I took salsa lessons, and I am a proud and somewhat clumsy newbie at upcycling and repurposing furniture. Things like that. Things that really made me put my money where my mouth was. After all, aren't we all, at some point in our lives, upcycling or repurposing ourselves? You can't constantly opt out. At some point, you have to step up, stand up, and get moving.

I'm no stranger to being knocked down. I've been shoved to ground, held under thumbs before. Many times. If you live long enough and have a relatively calm, successful, and happy life, there are definitely people who want to knock you down . . . just to see you fall. It's naive to think otherwise. That's life. Jealousy exists, although for the life of me, I can't say I've had anything that anyone would ever covet. I lead a very ordinary, pragmatic existence, but someone must envy all that blahness, I guess. I've entered situations, either by choice or by mandate, that were designed for failure. Professionally and personally, I knew how to deal with those situations. I like to call it the "Let's see her wiggle out of this one" mentality. "Learning by fire hose" is not foreign to me. This was different. This wasn't a "put your big girl panties on and power through" situation. This wasn't someone making a poor decision (most of the time me!) and dealing with the consequences, intended or otherwise, of those decisions. This was new. This wasn't my career. This wasn't my relationships. This wasn't my reputation. This was my *life*. And, without being hyperbolic, this truly was a matter of life and death. I had never, ever dealt with this type of challenge before. I didn't have a clue about how to deal with cancer up close and personal. Thankfully, Clarissa Pinkola Estes, author of *Women Who Run with Wolves: Myths and Stories of the Wild Woman Archetype* reminds us how important it is to share our stories. She writes, "I hope you will go out and let stories, that is life, happen to you, and that you will work with these stories . . . water them with your blood and tears and your laughter 'till they bloom, 'till you yourself burst into bloom." Crank up that fire hose.

So, I was slapped. Shell-shocked, kicked to the curb, deer-in-headlights slapped in face. My defiant inner warrior princess rebuked, "Whatever." Slight side note: I mention "bitch slap" at the beginning of this chapter. Now, it's not my intention to offend. It's simply the overwhelming sense of dumbfoundedness in myself that spawned this reaction when I first heard the news. In true Kaye fashion, I went from overwhelmingly sad to fight-mode mad almost immediately. That's how I'm wired. Maybe I'm a "mother bear" or maybe the wolf is my spirit animal, but when wounded or threatened, I jump immediately onto a *fight* path when given the choice between *fight* or *flight*. I take a blow—to the heart, to the mind, to the body, to the ego—and I pick up the fragments of my shattered psyche and start wielding swords . . . most of the time, at the nearest available target. True to wolf spirit, I'm not certain

I've ever been truly understood. Wolves are misunderstood as aggressive, vicious animals who attack without provocation. In fact, wolves go out of their way to avoid confrontation. However, when threatened, they stand their ground. Wolves demonstrate a deep connection to intuition and instinct. The downside to all of this is that wolves can also demonstrate lack of trust. I have always felt connected to nature, but I haven't always learned more about it. Now that things were getting more personal, I decided to explore my inner spirit animals.

I've never wanted to fight anyone at any time. I don't particularly enjoy confrontation. Life definitely has a rhythm and an order which I crave, and confrontation upsets that apple cart. Like my spirit animal, and in true Amazon warrior style, I run in packs. Small, but loyal packs. Packs for life. But still, when I'm alone, I find it liberating. I'm okay with not being easily tamed or domesticated. I prefer doing things my way. I would need both: my wolf and my warrior. I needed to lick my wounds. I needed to sharpen the sword.

Back to the stark white imaging room at the breast clinic. Wrapped in tissue but trying to regain some composure, I attempted some semblance of pathetic fight mode. "So, now what?" was my immediate, flummoxed response to those talented imaging doctors and nurses, who had clearly experienced this rodeo before. Yet, there I was. Alone. And scared to death.

"More testing. We need to find the source of the cancer. It's like finding a polar bear in a snowstorm."

Now, I appreciate a great metaphor as much as the next guy, but I seriously needed answers. Source? Didn't we just establish there was a tumor? Whatdya mean "source?" Wasn't the "source" cancer? Can't we just go in there and take it all out and be done with this? This moment was when the title of this chapter was born. I went from victim to bitch in sixty seconds flat. Little did I know how little I knew. About any of this.

"Well, let's do what we need to do to get rid of this thing and move on," was the only logical, obstinate response I could muster amidst the tears and terror. I changed out of the stale green hospital gown. I would be seeing a lot of those scratchy drab things in the coming months. I could not return to work that day. It was a cold, January afternoon. Little did I know how 2017 would skid right off the path I had originally planned and straight off a cliff into uncertainty.

Blog Post: What Cancer Takes

A breast cancer diagnosis out of the blue takes a whole of lot getting used to. The beautiful thing is that breast cancer is one of the most curable of all cancers, so we just "get used to it." It isn't special. It isn't unique. Once everyone gets past the initial lightning bolt of, "Oh. She's dealing with breast cancer," the buzz fades and we're all expected to move on with life. Since my diagnosis in early 2017, I've had a lot of time for reflection and resilience training. I've had a lot of time to focus and regain clarity. I've had moments of the highest highs and the darkest of days in recent memory. We see all these empowering mantras on the t-shirts and coffee mugs: "F*ck cancer," "I'm a survivor," "Cancer doesn't define me," "Hope," etc. Yes, wonderful reminders *to keep our minds in bright and shiny places. Truth be told, there are just some ugly truths about what cancer takes from those who have it, deal with it, and hopefully come out of it, well . . . Alive.*

*Cancer **takes** your* physical body. *Pieces and parts are sliced into and removed. Needles penetrate veins to inject poison in order to kill a beast that lurks inside. I remember sitting in the cushy chemo chair, watching the "red devil" (as chemo patients call it) slowly trickle down the tube and thinking to myself,* I'm literally shooting poison into me. THAT is poison. Poison to kill poison. *It messes with your head, to be sure. At the same time these poisons are killing away the cancerous cells, they're also attacking what's whole and healthy and in fairly decent working condition in our bodies. Ironic, huh? Breasts are removed. Armpits are carved into. Scars make road maps across a once pristine landscape. Cancer will never allow your body to be the same again. It's time for a new normal.*

*Cancer **takes** your* mind. *"Going there" is easy to do if you spend time in social spaces where survivors commiserate, offer up advice, and just plain vent. This can be a much needed comfort when you feel alone in the process, but it can also lead further into the "what if" darkness. You hear complaints of side effects. You hear advice for overcoming side effects. You learn about warriors losing their battles. You hear stories of survivors twenty-five-plus years out. Every single diagnosis is different; there is NEVER a one-size-fits-all when it comes to any of this. Ease of mind, and taking it back from cancer, comes from* real *knowledge, asking professionals for advice, seeking out the most natural, holistic, and homeopathic treatments available, and* *relying on close friends and family who have "been there." I rely on these to steal my mind back from this bitch.*

Cancer **takes** *your* future . . . *but, only for a fleeting moment, if you allow it. There is the diagnosis, when the whole world as you know it stops. Then, there is the fear.* What stage is it? Will I die from this? What is my course of treatment? *Tests after tests after tests are run. Then comes decision time.* Surgery, chemo, radiation? Combo of some? Combo of all? What about holistic treatments? How long? Will I have any quality of life with this? What are the long-lasting side effects of all this crap I'm putting myself through? Will I grow a third arm? *Far more questions than answers, and suddenly everything took a back seat—to losing my hair, losing my mind, losing weight, gaining weight, chronic nerve pain, that never-ending guessing game of whether you're ever going to feel remotely close to human again for the foreseeable future. That's what cancer takes. To fight back, we find that elusive "new normal" we so often hear about. Define it. Embrace it. Celebrate it. Practice gratitude toward it. Every day. Everything else is just noise.*

Cancer **takes** *away your patience. I've never been a patient person. Ever. Ask anyone who knows me well. I'm not even remotely skilled at being patient. I encounter a problem. I explore solutions. I want action. Typically yesterday. Straight lines from point A to point B make me almost giddy. Needless to say, getting through breast cancer is a process. A long, squiggly, and oftentimes, backtracking, backbreaking, and rebooting one with roller coaster rides that literally make you want to hurl. Apparently, I'll never get "over" cancer. It's part of who I am now.*

From diagnosis to the checkered flag of treatment completion, it took an entire year of my life—and we can't forget all the aftermath. That's coming up. Through three surgeries, sixteen weeks of chemo, twenty-eight radiation treatments, and all the "recovery periods, it takes time, it takes patience, and it takes a toll. Hey! Patience is easy—when it's the only option you have. Maybe I'm more patient now? Maybe my give-a-crap meter broke a little in the process, but I see things through renewed perspective. It only took fifty-some years and a cancer blow to get that through my thick noodle.

While yes, cancer takes a lot, it **cannot** *possibly* **take** *everything.*

Cancer **cannot take** *the core of who I am. I was made crystal clear about this, early on especially, when Facebook posts, messages, emails, and cards from those who knew me best actually pitied cancer for being stuck with me. Wait. What?! While I'm sure these were meant to spread good cheer, I guess it says something about my inner badassery. At first, the posts made me think,* Ghheeeez . . . am I that intimidating? Really? *Turns out, it takes a ton of badassery to stand your ground against cancer. I had to dig deep to resurface that uncoachable, defiant, line-in-the-sand warrior princess who got me into trouble many times throughout my life. She absolutely was in there; just on hiatus, likely sipping Corona in the sunny sand somewhere because I just didn't need her as much anymore . . . until then. Determination, focus, and a HUGE dose of clarity ironically became gifts from this whole shitshow of an experience.*

Cancer **cannot take** *an irrepressible spirit to learn. I* *unabashedly love learning, and through all of this, not everything I learned was pleasant, but it was valuable. I learned quickly who my true friends were, who my acquaintances were, who the inspirational warriors and supporters fighting the fight right alongside me the whole way were. I learned for whom and what to make valuable life space. It's those people who have made me a better person. And, I thank them all with my whole heart.*

The thought that I could do it all, be it all, and have it all—by myself—was one big, fat lie. It's not easy to acknowledge. I've also learned to honor that little nugget of information and forge ahead, and graciously accept help when offered.

*Cancer **cannot take** the gift of new opportunities and doors opened from this nasty bout with a devil. Cancer, no doubt, delays things, but we have the power to consider what opportunity can look like once we've gone through this dance. Richard Paul Evans tells us, "It is often in the darkest skies that we see the brightest stars."*

I was repeatedly reminded that cancer patients actually found "good" in their journeys. Of course, my initial warrior princess reaction was a resounding, "You have GOT to be kidding me!"

But, I *see* it now. I *see* good. I *see* opportunity. I *see* light beyond measure for the remainder of my days, regardless of how many I have. And for that, yes. I am grateful for this god-awful life experience. Gratitude is something cancer cannot take. Ever.

I know now after listening to far too many stories of fellow survivors that it's incredibly easy to leap into guilt mode when you get a cancer diagnosis. *What did I do to get this? What didn't I do?*

Was it having kids early in life? Was it the not-nearly-enough servings of leafy greens? Was it environmental? Was it parabens in my cosmetics? Aluminum in my deodorant? Hormonal? Toxin-related? Age-related? WHAT, damn it! WHAT brought this on? I wanted immediate answers. They never came. As a matter of fact, it took an entire month and multiple biopsies, MRIs, ultrasounds, and lots of pin cushioning and scraping to eventually "find the source." That was one elusive polar bear!

That said, I never thought I'd ever shift my thinking or share this. I'd spent so much time thinking about what cancer had taken from me. Granted, I had my own polar bear in a snowstorm to find, and that was some feeble attempt at grace through all this. It's taken some time and some level of persistence. Through mindfulness practices, I found myself considering what cancer gave. The first gift is *clarity*. I see things that have eluded me for years, whether by choice or by circumstance. I had always thought I had a concise vision about how I wanted to lead my life. That was not the case. After cancer, the waters are no longer murky, and I find myself less frustrated and questioning less because I now have at least some of the answers I seek.

Humor. I pride myself on having a pretty strong sense of humor. There are instances when an audience can change that, but for the most part, I like to laugh at my foibles. I can be funny. I love to laugh . . . out loud. Obnoxious, embarrassing guffaws make me happy. Before all of this, I wasn't very good at laughing at myself. For whatever reason, I struggled with finding humor in my mistakes or lapses in judgment. I thought they were serious character flaws and annoyances that required immediate overhauling. Because cancer breaks your soul to some degree, there came a point when humor, and laughing at myself and my condition, filled the cracks in my soul that cancer had left. I tiptoed around like an elephant in a ceramics store trying not to offend others because cancer *is* quite serious and is an incredibly delicate matter. But for me, humor, albeit at times inappropriate or inopportune, helped me deal and helped me heal. It allowed me to salvage pieces of me. Humor glued the scattered pieces of my soul back together.

Focus. I tend to think like a squirrel who jumps from branch to branch. I can multitask, jump from one idea to the other rather effortlessly, and embrace the "abstract random" part of my personality. For a little context about learner types, "abstract randoms" prefer freedom over rules and busy, multi-sensory learning environments. It's neither a good nor bad classification; it just emphasizes the fact that we all learn in unique ways. Cancer, or any nasty challenge, demands every ounce of your attention in order to fully grasp its impact. Cancer helped me learn how to focus. I zeroed in on all critical information, resources, and strategies. While I am still keenly aware of my condition, I can readily shift gears and focus on one thing and see a task through from start to finish without being diverted by those pesky squirrels.

Compassion. Because cancer forced me to rely on others' concerns and offers of help when I was at my weakest, I now take my time reacting to someone else's problems. I came to see how judgy I had been, and this revelation stabbed me in the heart, to be honest. Funny how cancer has a way of making you see things through a mirror and not a magnifying glass. What made me question my own behavior was witnessing behaviors of others when I was first diagnosed. Some folks who had no idea what I was going through passed quick judgment. Again, I think it's just part of being human. And, to be clear, these instances were few and far between. The quick judgements didn't sit well with me during my road to recovery, so I refused to do the same to others. I refused to return to being *that* Judgy McJudgerson. Today, I find myself much more reserved, suspending the judgy trigger finger until I have a fuller understanding of an individual's circumstances. Again, it's still a flawed work in progress, but at least I know how I *don't* want to act and continue to work on it. Stephen Covey, author of "The Seven Habits of Highly Effective People," reminds us to, "Seek first to understand and then to be understood."

Gratitude. Every single day. Every single moment. Giving thanks for each blessing because there are so many from which to choose. Home, loved ones near and far, increased energy and strength, a fulfilling and meaningful career, the promise of a cure . . . just the tip of the gratitude iceberg. Sitting at the very foundation of this iceberg of gratitude is my partner in crime, my partner in life, Dave. He and I have been together since we were new-to-adulting teens. Through our years together, we have grown, we have swapped parenting roles, we have changed who worked outside of the home, and we have been afforded the luxury of a long marriage because we made a conscious choice to grow together rather than apart. Like most marriages, it takes a whole lot of effort. To say I'm lucky is the biggest understatement I've ever heard.

So. What *caused* this? It *might* have been stress. Type A personalities drink stress like Kool-Aid. That's all well and good, but

I flailed about miserably trying to find consistency in any positive stress management practices. Notice I said, *flailed*, not *failed*. Failure is only failure if you don't learn from it. I flailed about, jumping from yoga to sweat equity to calming teas to meditation/prayer to . . . you name it. All are positive and potentially impactful in reducing stress levels. Working on something consistently is at the top of my to-do lists. C'mon! Type A, remember? I need lists. I crave them. They're my air!

It *might* have been my weight. I'm a big girl. A strong girl. A sturdy girl. Always have been, and I'm damn proud of my strong, stable makeup. This Amazonian constitution has gotten me through many dire situations, and for that, I am thankful. I would need this robust physicality down the road, to be sure. "Good breeding stock," my wonderful mate-for-life husband said when we first began dating. He's good with flattering words like that! But I guess there's absolutely room for improvement. Another thing to add to my to-do list.

It *might* have been my diet . . . or lack thereof. Let's be honest. Kale, in all its healthy goodness, just doesn't always stack up to the mighty satisfaction of boneless chicken wings. Finding that balance of my love for all things green (sans kale, sorry) and rich homemade goodness of comfort casseroles is tricky, but necessary. Striving to add leafy greens to every meal is one small step in a positive direction.

It *might* have been environmental. Every day we are inundated with more and more chemicals and toxins in everything from cosmetics to the water we drink. Turn on the nightly news, and it's always something. Sunscreen is good . . . sunscreen is bad. Coffee is healing . . . coffee is harmful. It's shocking that we don't break our necks from the informational whiplash we encounter.

It *might* have been the fact that I do favor a satisfying, robust ale or wine spritzer. Could I have done without those festive events when the allotted one or two were not enough? Maybe. All of these, coupled with other hormonal nuggets and the blessing of aging, are factors in developing breast cancer. I underscore factors because, as I have now been made painfully aware, breast cancer isn't *caused* by any singular thing. It's a mysterious mix of risk factors that concoct this horrific perfect storm with hormones inside your body. And then, all hell breaks loose. Polar bears in snow storms.

The only thing you can do in this situation is shield up. Amazon warriors, princesses or not, can take a bitch slap. It hurts. They embrace the pain, they own it, and they punch back. Slaps are for sissies. Punches are for warriors.

Dear Kaye,

Thinking of you often, praying for you daily! You have always been a strong, confident, motivated woman! All of these things will help you through this difficult time. Keep on trucking!

Love,

J.G.

Kaye,

I just wanted to drop a note and let you know that I've been thinking a lot about you. From the looks of your FB posts, it would appear that you had a positive report card at your latest doctor visit. That is FANTASTIC news!

Prayers for continued strength, healing, and health are being sent your way. One's health is something that can easily taken for granted. Your courage through all of this is very inspiring, and I want you to know how much you ROCK!!

PEACE OUT, WARRIOR! You SO got this!

Always,

L.Z.

Chapter 3: Paralysis Mortalysis When You Face Your Own Demise: Mustering That Amazon Bravery

We are afraid of our power.
~Mary Williamson~

Being brave is for cotton-headed ninny muggins. Watch *Elf*. It was, and always will be, funny. Everyone deals with cancer news differently, and it's not always by being brave. I respect those who keep things to themselves. No one else needs to know your business unless you want them to. I started out that way. I journaled for my own sanity. I holed up in my house for days on end just to shut out the world, and I found sanctity in a safe home and work routine . . . and yes, dog cuddles with Geneva. At the beginning, I was so traumatized, I spent quiet moments trying to calm my thoughts. A close friend sent me a framed, 5x7 rainbow-colored piece of letter art that said, "Maybe swearing will help." Perhaps. I wasn't quite ready for disclosure. I couldn't lay all of this murky mushiness going on in my heart and head on Dave, though. Being a constant burden on loved ones wouldn't help anyone. So I kept everything bottled up for a while. It wasn't healthy for me. I had to find another path. It may have been a socially perilous path filled with poison arrow dart frogs and flesh-eating piranha of the Amazon by putting it all out there—telling my story—but it was my choice. My path. Warriors do that . . . and we don't look back.

Deer in headlights. Dave and I privately spent so much time wrapping our heads around the enormity of what was happening—basically, just getting through each day, hour by hour—that we forgot to actually live when we finally reached that precipice where every joint no longer ached and burns no longer required salve and gauze. This accounted for far too many situations when I couldn't react with levelheaded responses when people asked questions. For a period of time, I wasn't levelheaded at all. It's why I lost my keys, my grocery lists, even my large computer bag for work. It's why I skipped out on gym dates, social hours, and anything that would require clarity of thought. Paralyzed. That's when it dawned on us that living the remainder of our lives together would never be about money or things or prestige anymore. Headlights . . . with a rough bumper tap on the backside.

Because of the paralysis, I quickly realized that all that mattered was time and making memories during the time we have with ones who mattered most. Once you poke a few painful punches on life's time card, you're all of a sudden acutely aware of how many punches remain on it. Book the flights. Try the squid. Brave the ziplining. Attend the kids' band concerts or grandkids attempting to play the trombone for the first time. Watch them grow, and guide them through all the failures and successes they will inevitably have. Cultivate them to become thoughtful, resilient, compassionate people. Be there for your kids and enjoy them, regardless of age or geography or lifepath. Not everyone gets that opportunity. Make those time card punches count.

Cancer forces you to dig deeper into the thinking well. We don't ever want to go there, but it's a harsh truth that there is *no* given when it comes to time on Earth. Find your tribe. Embrace your people. Love them fiercely. Defend them in true warrior princess fashion. They need you, and they're awesome. Sip the wine. Take salsa dance lessons. Laugh your face off. This is what true bravery is.

Like I've said, it just wasn't fair to lay all of this on Dave. So, I journaled. Sometimes to deal with my fears. Sometimes to ponder questions that consumed my thinking. Sometimes to vent. Sometimes to record dreams and happy thoughts. Looking back, journaling was a lifesaver. I firmly recommend it to anyone going through anything—a place to count blessings, a place to air out frustrations, a place to record dreams and aspirations, a place to expose fears . . . and hopefully provide some reflective tools needed to deal with all of these. It doesn't have to be fancy. I thought I had to purchase some brightly-colored markers and an oddly pre-populated journal. I found it all complicated and distracting. A comfortable pen and spiral notebook would suffice, as would my trusty laptop.

Journal Entry: February 2nd

Manifesto \, ma-na-ʾfes-(,)tō
: a written statement that describes the policies, goals, and opinions of a person or group

: a written statement declaring publicly the intentions, motives, or views of its issuer

I'm never going to be the same. Already, I see a change in my thinking, a change in myself. Soon there will be a change in my physicality, which is the least of my concerns. I just hate, with my entire being, this cancer . . . and ALL cancers in my life. I want them gone, eradicated—forever.

I'm never going to be the same. Maybe that's for the better. Maybe I'll learn moderation. Maybe I'll learn to forgive myself more readily. Maybe I'll learn to forgive others. Maybe I'll eat more fruits and veggies. Maybe I'll stress less and love more. Maybe I'll learn how to drive back the urge to stomp the shit out of anyone, anyone, who hurts my family. Maybe.

Floodgates of memories open when I revisit this entry. I lugged around so many angry elephants on my shoulders at the beginning of this journey . . . even before this journey. Even as time has passed and healing continues, I still find myself overcome with emotions where reaching for my journal would have been the best first step. They just hit at the most unpredictable moments. It's funny how your own thoughts can be healing, though, and even humorous at times. I was scared. I was angry. I was paralyzed. Anger is heavy. Anger is dangerous. Anger can cripple. Anger can also make you sick, physically and emotionally. Anger is cancer.

Remember that Cancun trip that absolutely, unequivocally needed to happen, come hell or high water? Or a radical, bilateral mastectomy? Both weighed heavily on our minds. One we anticipated with childlike eagerness on a Christmas morning. One we anticipated with dread mixed with a smidge of hope to end all of this. The seesaw dichotomy of these two events was paralyzing.

Journal Entry: February 16th (on the flight returning from our Cancun trip—almost four hours of think time. Whoa!)

Returning from seven days in Cancun. Seven days to not think about work—yeah right. Seven days to not obsess about whether my family was okay—not happening. Seven days to not think about breast cancer. Um, no. What did work, though, was a much needed reconnecting with Dave. We walked the beach every day. We shut our phones down and dumped the Kindle readers. We drank Dos Equis and played pool games and horseshoes. We met new friends from foreign places. We ate really good cuisine—a lot of it. We worked out in a beautiful infinity pool every morning. We talked, and cried, and talked some more.

We talked about what kind of shark tooth to get B.D. We talked about whether A.M. would like a purple or realistic black and white orca whale. We talked about what size shirt would best fit K.D. We talked about what a great idea getting our cell providers' Travel Plan (international minutes) was so Dave could get birthday wishes from Ashley, Jordan, and Sam. We talked about how lucky we were to have Robey and Michele caring for the dogs (we had three at the time) and watching the house and how much our rescue princess pooch, Geneva, must (hopefully) miss us—or maybe it was the other way around. And we talked about the cancer and what was in store for us when we returned.

We didn't do much adventuring out this trip. I think we spent more time venturing in. I know I spent a good deal of time lost in thought, as the rhythm of the ocean waves pounded the shore. We did A LOT of people watching as well as listening to all of the different languages being spoken. We met friends from Argentina, Virginia, Canada, and, of course, it's easy as heck to spot a cheesehead in the crowd.

For me, this trip was more reflective and preparatory therapy. Some cancer patients seek counseling; my counseling seems to come from nature. An important topic we discussed was setting a few easy changes in lifestyle goals once we returned: (1) walks every day (inside or outside), (2) more fresh juice—we fell in love with a healthy "green" juice here and got the ingredients list, and (3) limiting processed foods. To infuse some humor into the therapy, we set some silly travel goals for the next vacation: (1) Speedo Stephan and Bikini Bertha (don't ask), (2) shorter than seven days (I think we both got homesick), and (3) pack lighter and smarter (yeah, that's mostly me).

Then, we readied ourselves for returning. Tomorrow (02/17/17) is the big consult day. We meet with the plastic surgeon who is doing my reconstruction, and then we meet my breast cancer team. We should walk away with a more definitive plan so I can arrange work (and life) schedules accordingly. After all the testing and not knowing what exactly we were dealing with, not being able to schedule events a month and beyond has been super frustrating and rather stressful. I love what I do, and the thought of not being able to do it really bothers me. Not knowing how much I will have to lean on my colleagues is incredibly

*frustrating. I don't like being dependent on anyone. One thing
I'm slow to learn is that I don't get to control ANYTHING in this.
Nothing. That's not an easy pill for a control freak to swallow.
But I'll get there . . . maybe.*

To battle paralysis mortalysis, I spent a great deal of energy
inside my own noodle, processing and gaining perspective,
trying to make sense of everything and engaging in a hefty dose
of positive self-talk. That's neither healthy nor harmful. My job
would not be affected greatly. *Come on, Kaye! Get real.* The work
would absolutely be there when I was ready to jump back in full
throttle. Thinking big picture was a stretch at that point. All I
could see through my cancer blinders was the "right here, right
now" scenery. Even tomorrow seemed distant at the beginning
stages. It's natural for those thoughts to clang loudly when you are
entirely committed to the work, the purpose, the momentum, but
I was entirely ill-equipped to grasp much, if any, rational thought
at the moment. I was getting closer to revealing my deep, dark
secret to the world.

Then, there was this issue of hair loss. Many women going
through chemo for breast cancer will testify that this is one of the
most impaling side effects they experience. That loss of femininity.
Loss of perceived beauty. I get that. Thankfully, losing my hair
ended up not being a big deal for me. Really. Think about it. I
traded mornings of taming down some gnarly bedhead, pasting
on product, and stressing about the amount of gray I needed to
cover for mornings of wash, pat dry, cap or scarf, and out the door.
Easy. Five minutes tops. I even had time to make some fun little

protein-rich snacks for breakfast. Food was not my friend during chemo. Nothing tasted appealing. Hair loss ended up not being overly concerning.

Learning to accept the loss of a physical piece of me that had pretty much defined me since I was in the fifth grade? Also not a huge deal, for the most part. I worried more about Dave than myself when it came to losing my breasts. I had to deal with them since fourth or fifth grade. I had to duct tape them during a track meet so they wouldn't flop around when I was running my races. No joke. I had to pay stupid amounts of money to find the right sports bra to support the top-heavy buxomness. He adored them more than I did. Naturally, his feelings mattered more to me. We had long discussions, most of them uncomfortable and awkward. You would think that after more than thirty years together, there would be no more of those. Yet, this time I *really* needed him to be honest about how he felt about this particular loss. It was his loss, too. What it boiled down to was that yes, they *were* integral parts of who I was, but they were physical parts. And now? They were potentially killing me. Thankfully, we agreed. They had to go. It made me think about those Amazons again. If they really did cut off one breast to improve their marksmanship with a spear, what went through their minds? Did they "take one for the team" for the sake of winning the battle?

Time to put on a brave face. Have some positive self-talk time: *chemo and/or surgery and/or radiation won't kill me, right? I'm strong; I'm sturdy. I'm an Amazonian. A warrior princess, remember? I will grin and bear it.* Okay. Maybe not grin, but people do this cancer thing all the time . . . and for much longer treatment periods than mine, right? No big deal. Talk about an exercise in pure senselessness. It was almost mandatory that my colleagues know. It became painfully obvious to me that I was not going to be involved as much as I had hoped on collaborative projects and timelines since my current timelines just got shot to hell. The thought of being inadequate and not contributing to the progression of projects was devastating. My job didn't define me, that I knew, though I took great pride in what I did. Although reassurances abounded, I have to admit—I struggled with this little thorn.

What ensued was learning the "cyclones of chemo," as I dubbed them. The two-week cycles of highs and lows that accompanied each treatment. I learned about cumulative fatigue—I'm not talking the, "Gee, I could use a nap" fatigue, either. This stuff is for real. I experienced "Steroid Saturdays and Sundays," when I thought I was Wonder Woman, and I navigated through points in the two weeks when I clearly should not make critical work/life decisions. I learned to listen when my body said everything would be just peachy to go ahead and give 100 percent and when it would clearly be a negative 50 percent, not happening, head-in-covers kind of day. I learned that there were always more "better" days and how to honor the time needed to rest and regroup to face the next cycle.

Then, there are the personal struggles, the deeply private ones. The ones that cut deeper than any scalpel ever could. The ones when tears flow when all alone. I'm not terribly fashion-forward or overly concerned about whether my socks even match most days, but when you go in the closet and take a look at the beautiful, buxom-fitting Victoria's Secret® pretties, knowing that you'll never wear them again, that's a bit of a dagger. A bigger one than I had initially thought. Then, there's the whiplash that catapults you into apathy. How awful is it to not even care? About anything? It rips me apart to recall the days I didn't care whether or not I changed my underwear, much less care if it was pretty or matching. There were days I didn't shower. There were days our home was a complete, FEMA-certified disaster zone. There were social dates I avoided, postponed, or downright canceled. The kicker was that this passionate, wild-eyed, fire-and-fury wolf-spirited warrior princess could not have cared any less. I *did not* care. And, I didn't care that I didn't care. That was 100 percent not me. At all. Apathy has never been in my vernacular, and it drives me batty when I see it in others. All of a sudden, this apathy thing was my reality . . . and I didn't care. At all. For me, it was just another dagger no one told me about. And, I don't care how Amazonian you think you are, or how fierce you think you are. Chemo, multiple surgeries, radiation, and everything that follows all take their own sadistic, grueling time with you in their respective torture chambers. I'm not ashamed to admit that I was paralyzed for a long time, entirely content with my hermit status. I was shattered—physically, spiritually, emotionally. No one needed to see that. And seriously? I just didn't care.

In the long run, I couldn't handle keeping it bottled up. I grew so, so weary of being paralyzed. Paralyzed with fear. Paralyzed with the unknown. Paralyzed with doctor appointments. Paralyzed with tests and more tests. Paralyzed with my own mortality. You wouldn't think sitting still and not going out much would only lead to more energy, more strength, more stamina to get through a normal day. You'd think. I'm certain I don't know anyone who sits around intentionally thinking about how long they will live. I never did that. Ever. Live life! Livin' la vida loca, baby! It's the only one you have! Life is short! YOLO. Life is unpredictable. All that positive LIVE, LOVE, LAUGH t-shirt and coffee mug mantra fodder. We all get it, but not once did I ever fathom the morbidity of pondering my impending doom. Until this. Sometimes reality just sucks.

Journal Entry: March 3, 2017

I won't lie. I'm scared. I'm anxious. I'm impatient. I'm distracted. I want to spend as much time as possible sheltered at home. Away from people. I wake up in the middle of the night in a panic. Once lucid, I can't recall the exact cause of my terror. Some nights, it's work. Some nights, it's the kids. Some nights, it's fear of what's to come. Some nights, it's imaginary boogie men lurking and looming outside in the yard.

Point is—I'm discombobulated. I'm disoriented. I'm dysfunctionally adequate. I'm in pieces, and I haven't even been sliced into yet. I want to scream. I want to punch. I want to sob. I want to kick. I want to cave. I want to crumble. I want to live.

Physically? I think I'll be okay. I'm a big girl. I'm strong. I'm fluffier than I should be, but I'm solid. Once the drains are removed and the wounds start to heal, I should be okay. Then, there's treatment. Treatment's a whole other beast. For someone whose medication intake maxes out at a couple of ibuprofen once in a great while, I'm so intensely fearful about what chemo and radiation are going to do to me. Killing cancer is one thing, but purposefully killing off the healthy cells? The drugs might end up being those boogie men, after all.

What if *how I feel interferes with my work, work that I love doing?* **What if***, in the absence of healthy cells, another type of cancer grows?* **What if** *I debilitate myself permanently with my hermit status?* **What if** *I revert back to my comfortable, safe, sedentary life?*

That's where I struggle the most—my mind. It's a true dichotomy. There are times I can move mountains with sheer will. Then, there's now. Bursting into spontaneous, combustible bouts of tears triggered by sadness, grief, fear, or frustration . . . or a combination of them all. My mind was convinced, at one time, that I was invincible and just did things because I felt like it. Now, I find myself cowering to the fear. I put on a brave face, but inside, I'm crumbling.

So, how do I change this? How do I get the stubborn, obstinate pitbull back to fight this? My logical self gets and analyzes all the data available—the facts. Knowledge gives me power and comfort. What I need to do is enlist that headstrong bitch on my weakest days. I need her when I'm puking my guts out. I need her when I encounter phantom back pain, once caused by my 40DDs . . . that are no longer there. I need her when my thick, straight as straw head of hair is reduced to a shiny dome. I need her to get my ass out of the chair and out on the road or elliptical. I need her to put the weights in my hands and guide me back to my once-toned arms. I need her to help remind me of my goals, to-do lists, and dreams for the next fifty years. I need her back. I need that fighting Amazon warrior princess back. I know she's in there;

I think she's actually been hibernating in preparation for this battle of all battles.

So, in a week, the first phase will be done—removing the cancer. Focus on the positives:

- *No more cancer*
- *Less weight on my shoulders and back*
- *A new lease on life*
- *An opportunity to be better*

Getting better. I've got some nasty habits to conquer and change. There are a few parts to my plan to eliminate them. First, there's TV time. I can have TV if I'm moving—and only if I'm moving. Next, I need to return to music—play playlists while walking, while lifting, while moving! Also, I need to lay off of the salt and try other spices for flavor. I should drink even more water. I will stick to microbrew, dark beer, or locally-made wine, and set limits. Oh, and I need to go for green . . . lots of green. Eat mindfully. Savor each bite and smell the food. Eat slowly and fill up faster. Enjoy time on food prep for a busier week schedule. Be present. Be conscious. Step back from mindless tech time. Try to keep moving. Reward myself with TV at 7:00 with Dave if I moved enough that day . . . and our dog, Geneva. Don't allow work to overwhelm. Learn how to prioritize and delegate. Allow ME time—meditate, work out, sweat, cleanse the toxins. I don't have a choice anymore. No choice. Live . . . or cave in and die. Check that. I DO have a choice—CHOOSE LIFE!

- *Choose optimism*
- *Choose strength*
- *Choose faith*

- *Choose drive*
- *Choose beauty*
- *Choose tenacity*
- *Choose charity*
- *Choose sweet equity*
- *Choose friendship*
- *Choose laughter*
- *Choose joy*
- *Choose humility*
- *Choose love*
- *Choose LIFE*

Journal Entry: March 4, 2017

T-minus forty-eight hours, and I cannot believe the level of anxiety I'm feeling. I know what to expect; I don't know what to expect. I think I'll heal quickly; I fear being laid up and weak for too long. I know that my prognosis is positive; but what if I die? What if I don't make it to retirement? What if something goes awry during surgery? What if they find something somewhere else? Who will take care of Dave? Just too much time to think, too much time to read about others' experiences, too much time to wait.

I'm packed for the hospital.

I have all of the bills paid to date.

I'm almost done with work emails and meetings and prep for when I'm up to returning.

The house is fairly clean.

There's gas in the car.

We've got meals prepared and frozen for the next few weeks.

I've taken some final "before" pics of the girls before I say goodbye. They've been with me for fifty years, after all.

I'm grieving.

I'm scared.

My heart breaks for Dave. He's had to bear the brunt of this emotional hell. One minute I'm optimistic and confident everything will be just fine. The next minute I'm a pile of melted marshmallows. I've paralyzed myself with facts and fears to the point that I find myself self-medicating with endless hours of mindless TV bingeing. I've convinced myself that all of this will be remedied once I've healed. It has to!

Everything I've read indicates that moderate exercise will lower the likelihood of recurrence. Maybe what will work is fear this time—bottle that fear and use it as motivational fire.

Motivational fire:

- *Devote thirty or more minutes every day to sweat equity—every day*
- *Close out each day with journaling and/or meditation*
- *Eat for fuel only—you can't get too far with water in the gas tank of your car*
- *Perky boobs need tight abs and toned arms*
- *Learn to say NO*
- *Eat mindfully—pause and savor*
- *Walk the talk, then put it all together to educate and inspire*

See what I mean? I share my journal and blog entries in their flawed entirety. When you get whipped around on a Tilt-O-Whirl of adversity, your mind goes pretty much sideways, well, all of the time. Journaling helps me purge my thoughts, no matter how nonsensical they seem upon reflection. Purging the negative helps leave room for positivity and much needed breaths of fresh air. Truth be told, I was journaling before journaling became a thing.

Immediately following surgery, we had a constant flow of visitors in our home, and we cherished every minute, even if I wasn't at my best. Again, enter the apathy of not caring what I looked like or how I smelled. I did come to adore a pair of red flannel Eddie Bauer® bottoms. For some reason, I associated them with serenity and healing. Still do. Guests traveled to our woodland residence, clearly out of anyone's way, to share comfort and well wishes. It meant the world to us.

During one of my conversations with a sister survivor who had reached out to me, I told her that I wasn't accustomed to all of this attention. Don't get me wrong. I like it, and sometimes I earn it for doing wild or crazy or comical or just downright pea-brained things. That was all good fun, something to poke fun at during the next social gathering of witnesses to said stupidity. This was different. It was foreign to me, and frankly, I had had enough of foreign feelings. For a huge chunk of my life, I'd always been pretty independent and did things my own way. Mostly out of necessity, but I had grown habituated to living this way. It was not always pleasant. It was not always easy. I learned a lot of life lessons after being slapped on the wrist a few times. I also learned how to fend for myself. It's the warrior princesses way, after all.

I also explained to her about how I just wasn't used to the sudden influx of well wishes, the cards, the gifts, the private messages on social media, the emails, the texts, the voice messages, the meals, and all the LOVE. I'd never received such overwhelming love. I guess I wasn't cognizant that much love ever existed, especially for someone many of these people hardly knew. Maybe it had always existed, but I had never allowed myself to actually *feel* it before now. Don't get me wrong. I feel loved by my friends and family, always have, but when you are fortunate to have a life filled with the freedom of living comfortably and doing for yourself, you ignore the fact that you just might need a little help (and maybe a hug) once in a while. This very wise and wonderful survivor told me something that resonates to this day: "Shut up and open your arms." That's t-shirt mantra material, people! She was so right. She also laughed and told me not to worry because all that attention and well-wishing fades after a while. It was at that precise moment I stopped whining about being grateful and did what I was told. Talk about a transformative pivot.

Enter paralysis. Fear. Constant fear. Whiplash moment after whiplash moment. Fear is a wonderful paralyzer. I feared every new ache and pain. I feared hopping on a plane because I might expose myself to all sorts of foreign agents and germs and maladies. I feared enjoying a beer. I feared going into large crowds. I feared going out in the sun, not going out in the sun, relaxing too much, not relaxing enough. Every move I made built a wall of fear in me. Brick by brick. Did I go too far on that hike? Did I lift too much weight moving furniture or hauling bags of dog food? Did I sleep the wrong way and jeopardize my sutures? I convinced myself that every phantom pain was something much bigger. I was paralyzed. I'll admit—fear kept me stuck for a while. It was, I'm sure, difficult for friends and family to fully make sense of. *You're done with surgery and treatment. You should be able to do more.* I'm sure I disappointed them. I know I disappointed myself. Enter the vicious apathy cyclone again. *You have no control, so why bother with anything?* And further into the paralysis abyss I fell.

What I have learned a year and some change beyond my diagnosis is that it's 100 percent human to visit the land of Paralysis Mortalysis. We all get scared. I still do on occasion when some wonky trigger happens, be it physical or emotional. Sometimes "what if" deafens all other attempts at logical thinking. I remember a quote on one of the chemo infusion room walls that read, "Don't go there until you get there." It comes to me often, when I get stuck, when I allow my thinking to dip into paralysis mortalysis. Anytime we're faced with life-altering adversity, we can go from zero to panic in a matter of minutes. It's like a constant, ominous dark cloud that hangs over our heads. This is all normal. Let's face it. Cancer makes you think about things differently. Sharp adversarial situations change our DNA a little. We're forever changed; there's no doubt about that. Channeling that inner Amazon warrior comes in handy. Get knocked down, fall off the horse, take a serious blow with a spear. The thing is, warrior princesses get back up, focused on the end goal: defeating the enemy. I would imagine they didn't spend a lot of time thinking about their own demise. They remained steadfast to the goal of victory, of survival, of thriving.

So, yes, it's pretty normal to visit. Just don't set up residency. Fear does not get the victory lap. I have to remind myself of this constantly.

I have to admit—this arrow hit me right in my comfort food bullseye. Yes! Magical!

Hi Kaye!

Just wanted you to know I continue to keep you in my prayers as you continue your cancer fighting and WINNING journey!

When I was going through cancer treatments, I found ice cream to be very therapeutic—magical emotional healing powers! (*smiles) Have a little ice cream treat on us!

C & S

Chapter 4: Screw the Roller Coaster Ride. This is Battle Whiplash!

You can never cross the ocean until you have the courage to lose sight of the shore.
~Christopher Columbus~

When I was first diagnosed, I was told repeatedly, "Kaye, this is going to be one helluva roller coaster ride." Nurse navigators are amazing. First of all, I haven't ridden a roller coaster since I was a kid when I puked all over my brand new Converse leather high tops . . . that I bought with my own money I earned working as a country DJ at our local radio station, thank you very much. I loathe roller coasters with all my being. Always have. Even watching them at amusement parks induces recurring fear and an insatiable urge to hurl. This one's no different. Nurses fill your bucket full of information, resources, and research—enough to make your head explode. It's all for the patient's benefit. I know this. They know what they are doing. No doubt about it. They hand you reams of patient information, all of which makes reading a Chinese menu child's play, assuming I have any Mandarin linguistic proficiencies, which I don't. Nothing makes sense. So you call them, most times inarticulate because what you're trying to ask is brand new and somewhat obscure, in a language—medicalese—you don't understand. They explain things in layman's terms and patiently reassure you that what you're going through is "normal." Nurses hold your hands, dress your wounds, tell you the truth, and ease your pain. I don't know how nurses do it, but I am wholeheartedly grateful they do. They do this day in and day out, propping others up to continue battling. Nurses are simply amazing. Maybe they are Amazon warriors, too.

With this incredibly amazing man beside me the entire time, we journeyed through what we have since come to call, "The Year of Whiplash." I'm not entirely sure why, but milestones on this trek oddly seemed to fall on holidays (that we observed, anyway). "The Year of Whiplash" looked a little like this:

Day After Christmas: I absentmindedly find a mysterious pea-sized lump (and subsequently freak out in silence for the remainder of the year) while in the shower. Let me tell you, listening to your intuition is powerful practice. Trust your gut and check those tatas!

Shortly After New Year's Day (which has been a thorn in my side for a number of reasons, but that's another book): Diagnosis. Multiple tests, biopsies, and mystery solving to finally find the primary source of origin. As I mentioned before, this is when my imaging doctor stated after biopsy #4, "We're hunting for a polar bear in a snowstorm." Swell . . . I never was good at hunting. And I'm not fond of bears, either.

Valentine's Day: Sun and sand in Cancun because we had planned this trip way back in August the year before so we could actually afford to go, and by gosh, we were going! We go. It's a solemn saltwater therapy session before the storm. The day after we return, we have the surgical consult. We are doing surgery before treatment because at first blush, the affected area isn't that big.

St. Patrick's Day: A day I normally adore because when else can you drink green beer and sing Irish songs without looking weird? Surgical pathology comes back. It's much bigger and much more aggressive than initially thought. More tests to see if the cancer has metastasized elsewhere. No green beer today. No singing either.

Easter: Surgery recovery feels great (ish). Chemo has begun; clumps of hair find their way down the shower drain. Take it all. Dave is my barber. Dog shears will do.

Memorial Day: My favorite season begins—Camping Season. Lo and behold, chemo takes a toll and even a campfire becomes dangerous territory for germs, infections, and potential delays in treatments. We see our beloved campsite and neighbors only three times this summer. Spend most of June sick, with a horrible summer infection and highly compromised immune system. S'mores will have to wait.

4th of July: Last chemo coming up. I can start feeling normalish again. My hair will eventually return. The anticipation of not requiring multiple daily naps is a beautiful oasis on the horizon. Yet, I still can't make it through a holiday weekend without a nap . . . or a gallon of sunscreen . . . or fear of campfires and mosquito bites. I'm asleep before any fireworks.

Labor Day: Fully recovered from a second surgery, hair is returning, and the realization that life is just too short as we learn about more friends and acquaintances burdened with this horrible disease. It weighs heavy on anyone's heart, but especially so when you're walking a parallel path with them. Radiation starts soon.

Halloween: Two weeks remaining in a twenty-eight day radiation regimen, and I hit rock bottom. The burns are blistered and purple. Any touch—clothing, moisturizing creams, a gentle shower—excruciating. I can, without a doubt, attest to the fact that this is the worst pain I've ever felt. Giving birth to a prickle of porcupines without pain meds would have been easier. Dead serious.

Thanksgiving: So many reasons to give thanks. Family and friends together, either in person or through the blessings of technology. Meals made with love. Food is somewhat palatable again. Weather allows travel. And health. Good health, physical and emotional health, for all! Blisters have healed. Scars begin to fade. Insides begin to regulate. Blessings beyond measure.

Christmas: The one-year anniversary of the "discovery." Sensing some stability for the first time in a year, only to experience the "aftermath." Treatment continues as does the dealing with a much more compromised physical being, mindset, and immune system. Adjustment continues. The ride isn't over yet.

New Year's Day: New Day, New Year, New Me! A year that is divisible by six. YES! Long story, and I'm not what one would call a true numerologist, but life events have taught me that so many good things and people are connected to the number "six." Looking forward with increased energy, increased enthusiasm, increased desire, and increased dedication to realigned priorities.

It's still a roller coaster at times. Battles are just that: roller coasters. To this day, there are still highs and lows, lulls and intensity, more good days and fewer not-so-good days. The cancer whiplash has, for many of these days, subsided. Peaks and valleys remain, but overall, the ride still is jarring but doesn't pose as bleak of a sickening and uncertain exit as it once did. We all experience times when we think we cannot forge ahead and raging fear is triggered again by the most innocuous event. There's that little voice we need to listen that tells us we're not done yet. There's more for us to accomplish. Listen to that little voice—it's intuition hard at work. We have more to offer, more to experience, more to feel, more to live. Listen to that voice. It's the voice of hope. It's the voice of purpose. During the last few days of radiation sticking with the mantra that "This too shall pass" was a tremendous challenge. It has served me well over my half-century-plus. I am not about to let it go now, but at times, it's hard. It's just so unfathomably hard sometimes. Keep hope alive. With hope, there is light.

Any warrior worth his or her salt never fights alone. Amazons certainly didn't. When you go through roller coaster, or worse, whiplash adversity, sometimes it's best to wave that white flag right away and accept those who want to fight it with you. By shutting up and opening my arms, I allowed more and more people into my once carefully guarded circles. I found my people. Not everyone will get Christmas cards, because frankly while it's the thought that counts, I'm not super stellar at actually sending them, but knowing that you have these support warriors in almost every corner you look around goes a long way to recovery and growing stronger and better. It is these people, precisely, who keep you from breaking your neck on that roller coaster ride. They are the ones who hold your hair back when you lose last night's mac and cheese. They are the ones who remind you how you became a kick ass warrior princess in the first place. They laugh at your mostly inappropriate breast cancer humor. They bring you scotcharoos when you need them the most. They send you Wonder Woman socks and chocolate. Lots and lots of chocolate. They are your tribe. Your circle. Hold them closely. Love them fiercely. Don't ever let them go. Without a doubt, your turn will come to return the favor one day.

When my wonderful nurse navigator, JoAnn, told me this would be "one helluva a roller coaster ride," I prepared myself (as much as one can) for that up and down, twisting and turning, hurling-at-the-end metaphor. Whiplash is different. Whiplash whips you. Whiplash breaks you. Whiplash takes longer to mend. Cancer is whiplash.

This note is one of my favorites and was shared with me on Mother's Day, a "holiday" that matters most to me. It tells me that our daughter is much like her mom (even though she will fervently argue this point). She articulates thought more profoundly through written word than spoken. I understand this. It was also accompanied by a coupon, handwritten by my grandaughter: "This is good for a ticket to the Overture Center with Momma." I love the Overture!

Dearest Kaye,

You are the strongest woman I know, and though it's hard for me to express verbal emotions, I thought if I wrote it, it would be much easier to convey. Everything I've learned about being a mother I've learned from you! Thank you so much for showing me what it looks like to be a caring and loving mother. A.M. says you are the best in the world!

You are my advice giver. My hand holder. My problem solver. My musical companion. My shopping buddy. My SVU aficionado. And my best friend!

My admiration for your strength grows everyday, and I love you more than any other. I'm so happy to have spent yesterday with you and excited about today! Along with all our tomorrows!

Love you sooooo much!

Ashley, A.M., and B.D.

Chapter 5: When Battles Wounds Hurt

{
One word frees us of all the weight and pain in life.
That word is love.
~Sophocles~
}

I'm not a hugger. Or at least, I never *was* a hugger. My parents weren't really huggers. I learned how to hug from Dave and my kids, ironically. How horrible of a parent would I be if I put them to bed without a hug? How awful would those first days of kindergarten, junior high, the last days of high school and college, sports victories (and losses), or relationships be without a hug? No hugging at their weddings? BAH! No hugging when they gifted us with crazy, healthy, and huggy grandmonkeys?

No. Freaking. Way.

Hugging my kids and my husband is amazing. It taught me a great deal about how much love is a two-way street. Hugging my grands and holding them in my arms is a gift straight from wherever your happiest place is. Take a sunny, breezy day in the seventies (no humidity or mosquitoes), the smell of freshly mowed grass, laughter, and mix it up with a pint of Ben & Jerry's® Mint

Chocolate Chunk . . . and that's what it feels like. If you prefer calling it heaven, by all means do. There is nothing in the world like an unconditional hug . . . until you can't. Then, it becomes going down a one-way street the wrong way, speeding and inevitably crashing into a light pole of despair.

I pride myself on having an obnoxiously high threshold for physical pain. I am not sure where it came from or when I first recognized it. It's just always been there. Maybe it's one of those warrior princess prerequisites. There were no medical advances in pain relief in mythological times. There were no OT or PT sessions to get limbs back in working order. Amazons often healed their war wounds with fire and cauterization. Herbs and alcohol were their pain meds of choice. They used what they had on hand and the wisdom of shaman to cope with pain. Oddly, I followed suit. I broke fingers in high school basketball and simply leveraged some mad duct tape skills to mend them. Hence the crooked pinkies on both hands. I gave birth without much medication. Trudging through a nasty sinus cold or influenza? Ride it out. Snapped hamstring like ripped guitar strings in a water skiing mishap on Father's Day? Back on the walking regimen in less than three weeks. I know. Obnoxious.

Reflecting on my youth, I am convinced pain was my closest friend. Something I sought. Something I needed. Something I deserved or earned. I even went through a phase that I now know is referred to as a "self-harm" phase. I was a cutter during my youth. There was something inherently blissful about the pain I inflicted upon myself. Disgusting? Perhaps. I know. Watching blood flow seemed to me like some ritual of releasing all of the demons that parasitically devoured my insides. It was anger, bleeding its way out of me. It was grief flowing out of me like a river.

I've taught students who have also displayed these self-harming behaviors, and I noticed some incredibly painful parallels, so I learned all I could about my own tendencies to find a trigger and eventually, a resolution to all the madness. It helped me identify and assist those students when I could, so there's the silver lining in all that senseless pain seeking. It's uncanny to me how this particular reflection circled back to me during my darkest, and most painful, hours. I really hadn't thought about it much, to be honest. Maybe it came up during one of my many "purpose" reflections while journaling. Maybe I was meant to go through a phase like that so I could truly empathize with hurting students. I really don't know. Needless to say, I no longer harm myself— unless it's an 80 percent off clearance rack calling.

There's a lot to be said about pain tolerance. I can put up with a lot. Broken fingers. Muscle aches. The occasional acting like I'm eighteen and then facing the sad realization that clearly I am not. Those are temporary and tolerable. Cancer is different. Surgeries cut into you deeply and leave scars that are constant reminders of what was robbed. Chemo poisons you and leaves your insides playing all sorts of games (that are not fun, by the way). At the risk of a TMI moment, I can't tell you how proficient I became at playing "Bowel Movement Bingo" on any given day during my treatments. It happens when your whole system is acclimatized to the occasional Tylenol or ibuprofen for pain relief, and then all of a sudden, you're pumping poison through your veins. Not an acquired skill I necessarily wanted, but it's a reality in all this. You just never knew on a daily basis what would happen.

It was at this point in treatment that something like a mourning process overtook me. For whatever reason, I realized that too often I didn't appreciate how fortunate I was until what I had was gone. Not that I was purposely ungrateful. I just got so caught up in the chaos of life, so busy hurrying from one day to the next, I forgot to stop and be grateful for all that I had. On a seemingly superficial plane, I didn't realize just how meaningful lingerie or a fairly symmetrical chest really were. *They're gone,* I mused in the mirror most mornings. During all the chaos of surgery-chemo-surgery, I very rarely stopped to think about the disfiguring, and ultimate transformation, that was taking place. I never really thought about what *gone* actually was because, well, I never really thought it would happen to me. Maybe when something as simple as a hug became a physical challenge, it sent my noodle into a tailspin of everything that was *gone.* The truth is, sometimes the most painful wounds are on the inside.

Gone isn't just some throwaway term or trite cliché used to define the absence of something. *Gone* is real, and it's enduring. And *gone* does happen to us. Randomly. Unexpectedly. On a brisk, early March morning. What's *gone* was *gone* forever.

The inconvenience of a hefty chest, the cost of pricey yet durable sports bras, the tops too tight because of "bodacious tatas," as my girlfriends dubbed them. *Why does my back always hurt? Why can't I just get a normal-sized sports bra? Why does no one understand why I literally can't run without a jiggling issue? And, why do they insist on being close neighbors with my belly button?* Ugh!

Then, one morning shortly after Labor Day, out of the blue, I stopped and contemplated what all those whiny ruminations represented. And, I stopped. Ruminating, that is. Because they were *gone*.

What I'm trying to say is that sometimes our mountains are most times best left as molehills. Those challenges. Those little things that morph into unnecessary issues. Maybe it's the toilet paper roll flipped the wrong way. Maybe it's bouncy rounds on the treadmill. Maybe it's the LEGOs® you just stepped on at two in the morning. Appreciate them. Savor them. Do it now, while you still can, before they all become memories of moments *gone*. And as you do, know just how fortunate you are to have it. Every annoying, ordinary, lovely bit of it. Sadly, someday you might just find yourself like I was that post Labor Day morning, standing in front of a mirror with nothing but memories of times gone by, physicality lost, femininity diminished, longing for the chance to wear the lingerie I spent all that money on, to gripe about nipples protruding due to the sudden chilly change in temperature, to feel somewhat like the woman I once was. Hugs would return. My femininity might be somewhat restored. But, my girls. *My girls.* Were *gone*.

During this particular recovery period, one of many on this roller coaster, whiplashy ride of cancer chaos, I read a lot. I fidgeted a lot. I prepared a lot for the pain I would endure. I managed a subpar "okay" rating through these new pains and scars and mystery movements. Chemo fatigue was still very present. I guess I had wanted it all to be "better" after that last treatment in July. Shows you that what you want and what you actually get are two distinctly different things. Recovery periods during cancer treatments are not really recovery periods; they are more like brief reprieves, or a retreat in the battle. Eventually, warriors have to jump back into battle. Crap. It was brutal, but I survived. Being "okay" was the top tier bar I set for myself.

Then came radiation.

I was *not* prepared for radiation. Not at all. I had learned all I could about the side effects of surgery, of chemo, of the aromatase inhibitor I had been prescribed. I consumed research and information like it was that pint of Ben & Jerry's® Mint Chocolate Chunk, only not nearly as pleasurable. Perhaps fatigued with information overload, perhaps too scared to learn more, I did *not* learn all I could about radiation. The first few sessions I thought, *This isn't so bad. A little sunburn. I've been through worse. Slather it with recommended cream. Wear comfy tops. Get ready for the next round tomorrow. Move on. Be done.* What no one, not one person in the radiology department or survivor who had been through this living hell told me was how horrible the burning would be. Perhaps there's a good reason for this. Much of what was shared was how much easier and tolerable radiation was than chemo. That ray of sunshine was prominent in my mind as I went to treatments every day. *I've got this. No big deal. This too shall pass. Only five and a half weeks. This too shall pass.* I burned until I got blisters. I burned until I turned purple. I burned until I bled. This was not the same blood-letting demon release I experienced from my days of self harm. Unequivocally, this was the worst pain I've ever experienced in my life. Physically and emotionally. In hindsight, it was incredibly short-lived. I only had twenty-eight treatments. I know so many people who have endured much more. How? I have *no* clue, but I would venture to guess their mentality is, "You do what you gotta do." My mentality, for a lack of better definition, was feeble and ill-prepared for this "temporary" pain. I grappled with myself excessively—mostly focused on the intense pain and not on the "it's all temporary/this too shall pass" maxim. Not sure why I couldn't wrap my noodle around that level of mindfulness and positivity, but I flopped and flailed like a bluegill on a boat floor.

I couldn't hug. Not my best friend, not my dog, not my children or grandchildren. No one should ever experience so much pain that hugs hurt. The reality of hugs being gone, my girls being gone, apparently, my pain tolerance being gone devastated me. It was a rough patch, to be sure. The moments that hurt the worst were when our grandchildren asked to play, something as innocuous as LEGOS® or a mild game of war with our giant, souvenir "Everything's Bigger in Texas" cards. It was torture to say no to bedtime stories because I couldn't lift them to my lap in the rocking chair or lie on my side under a flashlight in a bed fort. I had nothing to give. When our children needed some assistance, maybe with cat-sitting or changing out some furnace filters or a quick shopping trip for school supplies, I had nothing to offer. When friends and family near and far, geographically distant and dear, wanted to make memories together—go out for pizza, dance at a former student's wedding, take a road trip to a local craft shop—I had nothing. Nothing. Zilch. Zero. Nada. For a period of time, which seemed like an eternity, I could offer nothing. There is nothing so helpless, and borderline hopeless, in the world than knowing you have nothing to give. Nothing to offer. Worthless. Now, I was *gone*.

Nothing besides taking up space. And healing. Ah! I had to heal. I had to snap out of these doldrums. I had to get back on my feet and stick my nose to the ground like a bloodhound, pound out the kinks in my armor, and do whatever was necessary to heal. This wasn't me, and I hated it. All of it! I had to get back to being the obnoxious oversharer on social media. I had to get back to offering my two cents, whether or not anyone asked for it. I had to channel my inner warrior princess, and rid myself of this hopeless, helpless ninny that was squatting on my life space. I am not *that* person. I am *not* a cotton-headed ninny muggin. I am a warrior princess, damn it. A wolf-spirited wild woman. Where the hell did I lose myself in all this? Where had I gone?

With all the flailing and failing, the one positive switch flip on all this pain was that little voice in my mind that kept reminding me, "This is temporary. Only ___ treatments left." It was focusing, but often deafened by misery. The countdown continued until the final and twenty-eighth treatment. In retrospect, something I found exponentially helpful while trudging through an adversarial moment in life was simply looking at this last step being THE END. While it may have helped at the moment, reality hit: there is no *end* with cancer. Believing there is an *end* to cancer is a fantasy. Cancer is just something you live with for the rest of the days you are blessed with, in some way, shape, or form. I just wanted everything to be over. My mind was done. My body was done. And yet, I wasn't done. Not yet. So hugging would have to wait until my new girls transformed and these particular battle wounds healed, but I knew where the hugs would be when I returned.

See? Whiplash.

This encouragement was accompanied by a beautifully handmade treasure that remains on my nightstand to this day. I love it and everything it represents!

Kaye,

Sending you positive vibes and prayers for quick and complete healing. Your surgery came as a shock and reminded me of how special and talented and strong you are. Just wanted to send you a little mug rug that I made for you. It's a little mat perfect for your favorite beverage and a yummy snack. Lay it on a table next to you, and know that I think of you daily. I'd still love to see you sometime.

Stay strong. Know you are in my prayers!

J.W.

Chapter 6: Gratitude and Growth: Empowerment through Battle

{ *Winning isn't everything, but wanting to win is.*
~Vince Lombardi~ }

Every time Amazon warriors returned from battle, there were lessons learned. They discovered the hidden paths they could travel the next time they would ambush their foes. They learned strategies of distraction. They learned to adapt their weaponry.

I didn't know a lot of people who had faced cancer. I had a few family members who did, but they never really shared their experiences with me. Maybe I should have asked them more. Maybe I should have offered them more. Since I had stepped onto the path, I wanted to learn more. I have listened to, and cried with, dozens of survivors, regardless of their type of cancer. Believe it or not, each person had something positive that came out of their experiences. Somehow. Maybe it was a job promotion, maybe a newly discovered talent or passion, maybe a reconnection to loved ones, or maybe a sense of life balance that had eluded them for years. At first, I'll be honest, I was indignant. *You have got to be kidding me—nothing positive can possibly come from this!* I was going to get my body sliced into pieces. I was going to take poison through a needle. I was going to lie on a table and fry until I bled. Come on! The only positive I could find in the foreseeable future was being done. Not being *over* cancer. Being *done* with cancer! For good.

Even though it was hard to see the light at the end of the tunnel, I am proud to say I never once swooped into a full-range, flailing chorus of, "Why me?" I'm not sure why; it just never dawned on me as a sustainable coping strategy.

"Why not? You certainly deserve a pity party," said my friends. Yeah. Nope. Not for me.

I learned from bouts with some pretty heady, and at times unthinkable, trauma much earlier in life, it really does no good to host your own pity party of one. I tried that. Through my grief as a child and developing teenager, there were too-many-to-count times I had lashed out in anger. Hostile, writhing, futile anger. I saw it in my students time and time again throughout my teaching career. It is, however, purifying at that rare moment, to sob like an infant, curled up in the fetal position. And trust me, *that* happened. Is was not pretty. All told, it was brief. It was spontaneous. It was cleansing. To add to all of the irony going on during my cancer journey, the angry sobbing eventually morphed into gratitude. I can't pinpoint the exact moment of metamorphosis. When I became overpowered by emotion, I just let the waterworks go. I had never done that before. That's gratitude bubbling to the surface. Sometimes . . . and this comes from practicing daily meditations and gratitudes . . . the fact that I am so very fortunate to have the life I've been gifted, really, catches me by surprise to the point of tears. Hence, the tears of spontaneous gratitude.

Among the countless gratitudes in all of this is that we caught this beast early. What if I would have skipped my monthly self-exam like I usually did? What if I would have brushed off the "little pea" as nothing until my next mammogram the following year? When I think about my grands—to date, four of them—I instantly reach for tissues. I was able to hold them all shortly after they were born, and Dave and I had been afforded the luxury of developing a bond with each one in unique and rewarding ways. Being there for them is truly what I live for. I want to share my stories. I want to watch them create theirs. The list goes on and on, and I can honestly say that I had spent a large chunk of my life not paying much attention to the overflowing abundance of gifts in my life. They were just there, roaming right along with me as I attempted to make a point, take a stand, prove something out of nothing, really . . . when all that ever mattered were these gifts. I took them all for granted. Everything. I encourage us all to hit the pause button for moment. Take a deep breath or two, and let ourselves wrap our hearts around all the good in our lives. Look around. Rummage through scrapbooks. Filter through an old toy chest. Open boxes of memorabilia from days gone by. It all comes rushing back in a flood of gratitude, and seriously? It grounds you when you feel like you're smack dab in the middle of the cyclone's eye. The road of pity is an easy one to travel, to focus on all of the things that are "wrong," to focus on things and people who are of little consequence in the grand scheme of the universe. Trust me, in my past I had spent far too much time and energy on all of these.

It was pointless. I needed to be done with all of the waste. For that, I am grateful. Through opening myself to growth and gratitude, I was able to turn grief into passion, pain into truth, aggression into persistence, judgment into acceptance . . . all of which snapped me back to the harsh reality that not everyone on a cancer journey is afforded that blessing.

Much like the dear survivor who told me to open my arms (and subsequently shut my face, remember), I had to open my mind and my heart to healing. I could not, in any sense, let the fear of the unknown "what-ifs" have any power over taking my life back. I wish I could say it was easy. Struggle is never easy; it's necessary. I never had a problem being headstrong. Ask my family. I did, however, struggle with being heartstrong like a warrior. I wanted to be better. Immediately. I still do. Apparently, like most things of worth and meaning in life, it takes time. It takes patience. It takes focus. It takes commitment to self. Even at this midlife (let's hope) pivot, I can still say I'm a work in progress.

How do we start on a path of gratitude when we're dodging shards of emotionally draining glass every single day? Taking cues from others, I started my healing process of gratitude with baby steps. I got a five-minute journal that filled up pretty quickly. By focusing on things for which I was grateful on a daily basis, I couldn't head into a pity party tailspin of all my woes of the moment. Surprisingly, those powerfully brief five minutes set the tone for the entire day, and I was able to acknowledge the positives and dive into the work I was doing at the time without being distracted by all the "what-ifs." One intriguing revelation that bloomed from the whole gratitude journal commitment was that when I stumbled a bit and fell off the gratitude wagon, my emotions readily followed. Fear crept in. Uncertainty crept in. The "what-ifs" crept in. When we live a life full of gratitude, especially during the most challenging moments, there is absolutely no room for negativity. In my many conversations with survivors and thrivers, others sang praises of gratitude journaling, praying, mindfulness practices and the like, but I had to fall face-first in the mud to recognize its cleansing power. Gratitude trumps everything.

I also started blogging again. I had started and stopped so many times you'd think I'd have whiplash. This time, I had something quite different to get off my mind. I needed to be honest about my journey, and I found that space to do so through blogging. I knew it wasn't for everyone. I honor every survivor's decision for doing what's right for him or her. I have made so many new friendships because of this unintentional sisterhood, and many were reluctant sisters. They didn't want to share. They wanted to forget every minute of pain. That's what worked for them. I honor that. For me, telling my story was cathartic. It was healing. It was necessary. It felt good to let the sarcasm and mostly inappropriate humor fly. It was rejuvenating to own the not-so-awesome feelings of anxiety, grief, and fear. I felt one step further, an ounce more healed, every time I spewed my thoughts on my blog. For whatever reason, it gained steam and people began reacting and reaching out. That's where this whole "write a book" idea came from—two parts me always wanting to write a book, two parts others giving me permission (and encouragement) to get it done. Sometimes all we need is a gentle nudge.

Inadequate. I think we've all felt like we're "not enough"

at some point in our lives. I want to believe it's natural to feel that way on occasion. As the gifts and well-wishes and pans of scotcharoos made their way into our home and our hearts, I felt an unquenchable desperation to thank every single person who had been so kind and generous to us throughout the whole process. I was just so profusely inadequate in doing so . . . I still am. In an attempt to find an authentic, orderly way to express my thanks, I hand wrote thank you cards to anyone who sent a gift or stopped by for a visit. It was such a small gesture, but it was satisfying to let others know their thoughts and actions of kindness were impactful and appreciated. I also posted a few thank you messages on social media because, quite frankly, my hands hurt, especially with the neuropathy that was still going on at the time and still continues today. Neuropathy is no joke. Google it. What a pain—literally.

I love coffee. I love the art of storytelling to make connections. One of my friends, in one of her many wonderful attempts at raising spirits and providing comfort, shared this particularly compelling, yet brief story. When it comes to gratitude and growth, consider this:

You are holding a cup of coffee when someone comes along and bumps into you or shakes your arm making you spill your coffee everywhere. Why did you spill the coffee?

Well because someone bumped into me, of course!

Wrong answer. You spilled the coffee because there was coffee in your cup. Had there been tea in the cup, you would have spilled tea.

Whatever is inside the cup will be what spills out.

Therefore, when life shakes you (and it will happen), whatever is inside you will come out. It's easy to fake it, until you get rattled. So we have to ask ourselves, "What's in my cup?'"

When life gets tough, what spills over? Joy, gratefulness, peace and humility? Or anger, bitterness, harsh words and reactions? 100 percent your choice!

Feeling like we've hit rock bottom is precisely the point when gratitude can morph into growth. Growth, for me, came in unexpected areas. For the first time in half a century, I learned to forgive. I started cultivating forgiveness for those whom I had harbored disdain or contempt because of some long-held grudge. I refuse to excuse their actions, but it was during this mindset-shifting period that I realized they've already put negativity into the universe, and I didn't need to add any more to my misery. This journey taught me that those individuals simply aren't worth the time or energy—something I, for whatever reason, had not been able to fully grasp until now. The universe will take care of them. Because of growth and gratitude, I no longer had space for hatred or loathing. My energy was successfully diverted to healing, inside and out. I aimed all my energies on love of family and friends, love of animals, love of country, love of self. That last one took a little longer and a lot more diligence. Any and all heinous acts in my first fifty years were not going to detract from what I aspired to accomplish in the next fifty. I'll address this a bit later. I had to seek forgiveness and practice forgiveness. A firm believer, I leave everything to the universe, or higher power, or God. You can choose.

Growth materialized in learning how to trust again—mainly, myself. For a long time, I knew (and I'm still not quite sure how) something was going on inside my body, and it wasn't good. Perhaps intuition, but how could I possibly know without a doubt? I'm not a medical professional, so I couldn't quite put my finger on it. Something felt wonky with either vitamin or mineral or hormone deficiencies and balances, which led to lethargy that led to low energy, which meant not getting in the heart-healthy cardiovascular exercise, which led to more sedentary habits, which led to some questionable nutrition choices, which just kept up this vicious cycle to "Nowhere-Near-Wellness-Land." Ah! Throw in a mix of anxiety and borderline depression, and it all came full circle. I should have trusted my gut all along. My body, my being, was trying to tell me something. I passed it off as one of those "blessings" of aging and largely ignored it. Hindsight has this obnoxious way of offering clarity. Drat! Self love really is a foundation for everything, and however you practice or express that is so, so important. Now when my intuition speaks, I listen to it, I honor it, and I act on it. Trust your gut.

Growth came in increased knowledge and a craving to assuage others' suffering. By nature, I want to solve everything for everyone and make everyone I care deeply about never feel pain— ever. Well, that's ridiculous. I've learned that being an enabler is not super healthy . . . or helpful. Carrying around others' pain is something, quite honestly, I believe led me to this cancer. Because I had to literally allow my control freak to die with the cancer cells, I learned how to help and love and support. I don't need to have all the answers or make all the pain go away. I can just BE. I can encourage and support resilience. This was, and still is, a lengthy and involved growth process, but I have no doubt I am better because of it. I hope it never ends. With hope comes promise.

We're all trees in this process of dealing with adversity. We plant a seed. We nurture it. We watch it grow. Depending on the species, oak trees are twenty to thirty years old when they produce their first acorns. Even then, acorn production is not consistent from year to year. Similarly, growth after trauma takes time. And it's deeply personal. That is what I, as a wannabe thriver, need to understand. Once you're done with treatments, once you're done with healing physically, the emotional and spiritual healing follows. This is then followed by, with all of the planets in alignment, prosperity. We need to nurture our process. Along the way to full maturity, a tree can still provide shade, shelter, and beauty to others. We can do this, too, as we grapple with our unique growth processes and go lightly on ourselves. I will refer to this more in depth later with the "Triad of Wellness" because it's that important.

I am hopeful that as my healing and helping continues, so too will my growth in learning. I am a relentless learner at heart. Yes, I have been called a "know-it-all" before. The moniker once irritated me, but that's the thing with cancer. Little niggles don't carry the punch they once did. I frankly don't care how pejorative that term might seem to some. I'm a sponge. I want to learn as much as I can about pretty much anything I don't know about. I will learn more about cancers, all kinds of cancers. I will learn about actions we can take, both privately and publicly, to sustain one another. I will learn how we can inch closer to a cure. I will learn what's truly best for an individual when it comes to survivorship, nutrition, wellness, western medicine, and the importance of innovative and complementary treatments. I've learned not to be buffaloed by BS and believe everything that's presented as gospel, not only about cancer but pretty much any topic of conversation.

Warrior princesses were straightforward. They didn't have time for gossip when there was a battle for which to prepare. They were brutal and aggressive, and their main concern in life was war. Focused. Because of this battle I never asked for, I've become a much more critical learner about what truly matters and what doesn't. I encourage others to do the same. Be the driver of your own learning and learn as much as you possibly can . . . about everything. Be that oak tree. Grow, my friends. Grow!

Kaye,
Your treatments . . . tough.
Your spirit . . . tougher.
Your courage . . . inspiring.
Your courage and attitude are amazing! Praying for complete restoration of your health.
Sincerely,
J.W.

(I apparently have more than one incredible J.W. in my life. What a lucky girl!)

Chapter 7: Letting Go–Time for New Strategies

> *The best revenge is massive success.*
> *~Frank Sinatra~*

I'm a control freak, Type A, multi-tasker, grudge holder. Guilty. As. Charged.

A wickedly wise and wonderful friend once advised me not to be so hard on myself and let things go. Funny. She is hard on herself, too. Hello, pot. I'm kettle . . .

My grandchildren, the light of my existence, love the Disney® soon-to-be classic, *Frozen*. Well, let me tell you. Cancer slams you into full-on Elsa mode and makes you want to belt out, "Let it Go." Hey, Elsa is kind of a warrior in her own way. She might not have swords or shields, but she sure can blast your heart into ice. At the very least you'll have a cool white streak in your hair.

Suddenly, vacuumed floors and an empty dishwasher stopped creating extreme neurosis. Rumor mills, gossip galas, and listening to others' complaints about politics, foot fungus, and the weather failed to render any needle movement on my "give-a-crap" meter anymore. No more bemoaning how "fluffy" I had gotten in the past few years. Gone were the days of caring as much about freshly primped hair, age-defying makeup, or getting to the gym every . . . single . . . damn day. Don't get me wrong. One of the best things a cancer survivor can do (if able) is to exercise regularly. It simply fell by the wayside when I feebly attempted to get any sense of balance, strength, or normalcy back. I knew all of the "give-a-craps" would return at some point; it just wasn't my reality at that time. Walk. Whatever the duration. Whatever the distance. Walk. Whenever you can. Get outside if at all possible. Connect with nature and all its miracles. Creating the strongest, healthiest version of yourself is one way to combat it all. As far as facing adversity goes, a healthy mind and body go a long way!

Nature. Let's talk about this for a bit. I'm a big fan of camping. Always have been. Our relationship with the great outdoors has evolved over the years. In our earlier days, we camped for adventure. Pull out the tent wherever there was flat ground, and set up camp. Eat whatever we could cook over a fire. Manage through the rain, kayak the back waters, come home smelling like we swam in a chimney all weekend. Glorious! Even at home, our entire neighborhood is filled with nature. Deer, turkey, squirrels, and the occasional black bear are our neighbors. Our nearest human neighbor lives about a mile away. Paradise.

Interestingly, wildlife instinctively knows when threatening weather is approaching. The animals know to hunker down when they are wounded or protecting their newborns. They forage for food and will sometimes travel great distances for sustenance. They know how to survive. We can learn so much from these creatures.

I'll bet Amazons were attuned to their natural surroundings and used what was available for survival as well. I could definitely relate to these characteristics.

Nature cleanses the senses. For me, nature is healing for a number of reasons, not the least of which is that I gain stillness and serenity being in the lush outdoors. It also connects me to my breathing and thinking more so than the synthetic over-grunting I experience in a gym. A simple walk down our woodland paradise provides a healing opportunity to reconnect with my spirit. I had spent a lot of time inside, and I missed out on nature and its blessings a lot, which stunk because it was precisely the place I needed to be in order to let go of everything weighing heavily on my heart and mind.

Journal Entry: March 14, 2017

I ♡ LISTS

Let it Go:

- *Guilt*
- *Caring what others think*
- *Regret*
- *Anger*
- *CANCER*
- *Material nonsense*
- *Wasted time*
- *Worry*
- *The past*
- *Petty drama*
- *Jealousy*
- *Gossip*
- *Small-mindedness*
- *Laziness*
- *Judgment*
- *Poison in my heart*
- *Crap food*
- *Fear*

Hold on Tightly:
- *Love of family*
- *Friends*
- *Love*
- *Hope*
- *Attitude*
- *Ferocity*
- *Joy*
- *Drive*
- *Desire*
- *Faith*
- *Adventure*
- *Tenacity*
- *Focus*
- *Knowledge*
- *Optimism*
- *Strength*
- *Endgame*
- *Goals*
- *Smiles*
- *Curiosity*
- *Promise*

The thing is, all of the junk I once lost countless hours of sleep over—deadlines, budgets, "frenemies"—lost their grip on me. What once was worthy of getting worked up over didn't seem to phase me anymore. Piles of laundry got done. Deadlines got met. Weeds got pulled. Bills got paid. Gym bag gots packed. Elliptical got its love. Sometimes it just takes the commitment to living with intention as opposed to merely surviving that results in a shake-up of the priority list. I've noticed this in my work and social lives as well. At meetings, I witnessed other professionals completely "lose their shit" about what I'm sure were highly sensitive and critical issues. Before all this, I would often inject myself into the fray, joining the hysteria. You know what? None of that ever really amounted to any substantive change, so . . . fast forward to my post-cancer self. Not much crawls under my skin anymore. We do the work. We focus on the good. We do our best. The results will come. Change will come. Not sure why it took so long and something so unthinkable to get me to realize all of this!

One of the most profound learning curves for me throughout my cancer journey, and one that hopefully, the reader, will take away, is that you MUST TAKE TIME FOR YOU. Up until that point in my life, I never thought putting myself first was all that important. Only selfish people do that, right? Family first. Obligations first. Saying YES first. Grow that network. Get your name out there. Answer every email within twenty-three hours. Don't leave people hanging. Can do. Can do. Can do. But it was hard for me. Still is. I don't like to disappoint. And, I don't like letting myself think I've let someone down or couldn't complete the task. I've heard time and time again that you cannot take care of anyone else unless you take care of yourself. I heard it. I ignored it. I found it rather annoying, truth be told. I would get to that later. Now, I realize how foolish I was. Don't be me; don't be foolish.

Ludwig Mies van der Rohe once wrote, "It is not possible to go forward while looking back." This resounds with me. It should with you, too. It's so easy to look at our past, who we once were, all of the beautiful mistakes we've made. Anyone who looks back and doesn't accept how much their past, no matter how "bad" it was, has shaped them, is in denial. But what I've learned is, it's futile to think we can do anything to change the past. Take your head, smack it against a brick wall several times, and come out without a headache. Futile. So look forward. Now I'm not suggesting that you look forward in the glow-in-the-dark, moon-eyed, perpetually perky, "I'm so looking forward to . . ." way. That's not me. However, by all means, look forward. Not every battle is an easy win. Let go of the anger of defeat and learn from it . . . then move forward. Will you continue doing what you've always done because you've done it that way for years? Okay then. Expect the same results. Stifled by fear? *I can't try this new thing. I've never done this new thing before.* OR, *I've tried that before with colossal failure. I'm not doing that again.* Okay then. It's okay to have "never agains." Some of those are actually good ideas to keep locked in the trunk of the past. Just take a deep breath. Let the past go. It is important to learn. It is important to remember at times. Just don't dwell. Walt Whitman once said, "Keep your face always toward the sunshine, and shadows will fall behind you." Undeniable. Whether it's fear of pushback from others or a potential fall from grace, make up your mind. Youth expert Josh Shipp had a saying that came in handy when I was teaching fourteen-year-olds that resonates for me now more loudly than ever, "You either get bitter or you get better. It's that simple. You either take what has been dealt and allow it to make you a better person, or you allow it to tear you down. The choice does not belong to fate; it belongs to you." Two options—bitter or better. So simple. Focus forward, face the sunshine, and don't look back. I know I've mentioned it before: forgiveness of self is part of the process. You have to start somewhere.

In *Women Who Run With the Wolves: Myths and Stories of the Wild Woman Archetype*, author Clarissa Pinkola Estés writes, "There is a time in our lives, usually in mid-life, when a woman has to make a decision—possibly the most important psychological decision of her future life—and that is whether to be bitter or not. Women often come to this in their late thirties or early forties. They are at the point where they are full up to their ears with everything, and they've 'had it' and 'the last straw has broken the camel's back' and they're 'pissed off and pooped out.' Their dreams of their twenties may be lying in a crumple. There may be broken hearts, broken marriages, broken promises." When I first considered writing my story, I teetered back and forth about dredging up my past. To tell the stories of my youth—mostly wild, unruly, undisciplined excursions into stupidity. I pondered exposing the abuse I experienced. I, to this day, have difficulty understanding how I made it through any of that alive. I thought about sharing my challenges with weight control, body image, creative processes, and my uncanny intuition. Then, I stopped. While every experience that has led me to cancer might have made for some wildly entertaining non-fiction, I opted out. I came to the conclusion that I should heed the sage advice of Ludwig Mies van der Rohe. This is about a culmination of all of those events. Nothing compares. Nothing even comes close. And while every life experience—the good, the bad, and the borderline illegal—has afforded me an opportunity to learn, this one slammed me into a learning curve like an Olympic bobsledder into a wall. So sorry, but the juicy, gory, and somewhat dubious foibles of my youth will have to be exposed in other written works of mine. Another story. Another time.

So, let's shift back to this bugger called cancer.

I've never had cancer before. I never intimately knew what people went through until I walked in their shoes. I knew so many survivors with a variety of diagnoses, not just breast cancer, who avoided even saying the "C" word like the plague. It pains them too much. I'm sure it is harrowing. Looking back, I suffered unnecessary turmoil thinking I had or hadn't done something to *cause* this cancer. Risk factors? Absolutely! Cause? No. Google it. Find Mayo, Harvard, Komen—none of those reputable sources will point directly at a *cause*. A myriad of risk factors, some of which I did or did not partake in, but no *cause*. Ask anyone who is either currently going through the process or lucky enough to be on a "survivors" list, my guess is they would share the same sentiments. It *had* to be something we either did or didn't do. Constantly agonizing over what I should or shouldn't have done wasted unimaginable amounts of my time and energy. Time and energy I very much needed then to heal and move forward. Choosing instead to shift my thinking to the now and the future, I focused on the fact that I had indeed developed breast cancer, I was indeed going through a treatment regimen, and I indeed was going to do everything within my power to ensure I lived a long and healthy life from here on out. This required me to hold my tongue until I almost bled when well-meaning (or not so well-meaning) self-anointed cancer pundits felt compelled to pinpoint the exact cause of my diagnosis: "Well, you are overweight and over fifty; that's a cause. I heard aluminum-based antiperspirant is a cause. Maybe if you exercised more or ate more turmeric and beets." Cause, cause, cause. Anyone else feel the urge to punch? Yeah. My response is and always will be, while nodding politely, albeit snarkily, "Walk in my 2017 shoes, and I'll be happy to entertain your apparent vast wealth of expertise on the topic." Essentially though, I had to pull an Elsa and let any and all comments go. I had to let my past guilt go . . . all of it. I had to face the sunshine and let the shadows fall where they may. I had to learn from my battle with anger, pull out my warrior princess playbook, and prepare for the next one . . . because there would *always* be the next battle.

Blog Post: 12 Things I Stopped Doing Thanks to Breast Cancer

1. I stopped looking back.
There's nothing I can do to change what's happened in the past—good, bad, or indifferent. I stopped the vicious cycle of "what if?" I've taken what I learned, and continue to learn, and apply it to what I dream and aspire to be and do moving forward. Let it mold me; don't let it define me or burden me. It's done. It's over. There's no benefit in regret or wishful thinking. Figure out what needs to be done and do it. I figure I have fifty years left to antagonize the heck out of friends, family, and colleagues. Let's do this!

2. I stopped listening to and believing everything I was told or read.
I understand well-meaning advice. I understand the feeling of extreme discombobulation that accompanies a potential deadly diagnosis. It plays with your mind. So, I became a voracious, informed decision maker. I looked to reputable resources and gleaned knowledge from research, case studies, and factual data on my own. Just because it shows up in a news feed does not always make it so. Consider the fine print. And the source.

3. I stopped beating myself up.
We're all human. We all have moments of pain, doubt, fear, and uncertainty. Getting worked up about work or relationships

or body image or the weather, for that matter, doesn't do anything to solve any of the aforementioned maladies. I've learned to find peace in who I am, in my capabilities, and in my future. Sometimes it takes a magnifying glass and a sledgehammer to find miracles and mercy in ourselves, but they definitely exist.

4. I stopped closing doors.

I'm not a hugger. It's tough for me to accept praise, and in the case of this stupid diagnosis, support. I'm not used to being doted upon. Opening the door and allowing people in has helped me "un-Grinch" myself. I feel my heart growing each time someone reaches out with a kind word or gift of support, and you know what happens? Turns out that sentiment leads to paying it forward and seeking out those in need. Doors are now opening all around me, it seems. It's turning out to be quite the win-win. And . . . it's A-OK to hug now.

5. I stopped taking myself so seriously.

I used to think I was defined by what I looked like or by what I said. I used to think I was defined by my career choice. For a big chunk of my life I wasted moments in scathing rebuke over my appetite, my temperament, my knowledge base, and/or my skill set—or lack thereof. Not anymore. What you see is what you get. I know exactly what I want. I find ways to get it. If I don't know something, I'll discover and pass along the wealth of knowledge. And, I'm willing to make sacrifices for those aspirations. If that offends anyone, well, that's on them.

6. I stopped being a "fangirl."

Not exclusive to my field of work by any means, I see it occurring everywhere, especially in the network marketing arena: "Buy this latest and greatest item" (most times lacking any substantial evidence or data to back it up, mind you). I've noticed quite the uptick of self-aggrandization taking place in the land of social media. Follows, proselytizing, and "likes" are nice but never really appealed much to me. Just do the work. Get your hands dirty. Get results. I don't need someone telling me they're "networking" or "connecting" when the only connection is to boost their own bottom line. Give me meaningful, authentic conversations around a local, rich microbrew or chai latte (vanilla, please) that cultivate deeper, much more rewarding relationships any day.

7. I stopped giving a crap about animal hair.

We have three dogs and a cat. Two of the critters live predominantly inside, mostly because they run the place. I used to spend hours on end chasing them around with my Swiffer® duster or vacuum trying to keep up with their "golden flecks of love" deposits all over the place. Not anymore. Once a week, maybe, and if our guests struggle with being "loved," I'll happily meet them at a golden-flecks-of-love free location. That goes for dust bunnies and kid-smudgy windows, too.

8. I stopped "going there."

Cancer makes you think the worst at times—especially during the dark days. What if it comes back? What if it spreads elsewhere? What did I do to "cause" this? What didn't I do right? What should I do to ensure it doesn't come back? Who's going to care for my loved ones? How many years do I have? What if I don't accomplish what I want to accomplish? It's okay and quite human to tiptoe around the abyss; just don't jump in. It can be a long, and detrimental, climb out.

9. I stopped allowing space for hatred or irrelevance.

Vengeance is a bitch. Let's face it. There is no sense in letting miniscule-minded, narcissistic individuals have any leverage in your life. They mean nothing. They have no significance. They have no place but in a toxic dumpster of the things you've let go. Let the universe take care of them. Focus on the happy, intelligent, uplifting peeps instead. They make us better.

10. I stopped the "Yeah, but . . ." circus.

Most times, our biggest enemy is ourselves. We need to stop it. Putting up barriers (most of them dandy fairy tales, by the way) doesn't help. The "Yeah, buts" close doors (see #4). Not anymore. Instead of thinking "Yeah, but I'm too . . ." or "Yeah, but I'm not . . ." I've decided to take the advice I learned at one of my absolute favorite leading and learning events—Edcamp Summits. "Yeah, but" has transformed into "YES, AND . . ." from here on out, baby!

11. I stopped saving sailor talk for campfires.

I don't normally swear—unless I'm struggling up that last bit of 7 percent grade hillside on my walks, around others who regularly exercise sailor mouth, or cannot think of a better way to phrase things. I cannot even count the number of F-bombs I've dropped since my diagnosis. I've realized that being dumbfounded frequently finds itself flanked in F-bombs. I try not to swear around my mother, who would disapprove, but for precision and posterity, I let it fly.

12. I stopped being trivial.

Little blips in life are no match for battling a life-altering diagnosis. So there may be nights when I feel lonely, unloved, or disconnected. There may be days when my favorite pants don't fit. There may be moments when someone says something that sticks in my craw for days. It's all trivial. Nothing compared to being sliced into, poisoned, and burned—all to kill a devil. Note to self: Get over yourself, self. Be Elsa—let it go.

I often hear the adage, "Let go and let God," and I think there's something to be said about this. Whatever faith we practice, whatever higher power we praise, letting go, being grateful, and following the process can be instrumental in healing. Notice I never said, "Trust the process." I've had my hands compassionately patted and told this too many times to count. Forgive me, however flawed my thinking is, but I don't trust anything I can't somehow control. Besides, I find it terribly cliché. That's just me. It's part of my healing and development in all this. Yes, this is a process. Any healing is. I want a say in the process. I trust having options.

I'll be honest. One of the biggest challenges to "Elsa-fy" for me was #9—letting go of any negative feelings toward anyone I once considered a nemesis or yes, a downright enemy, to my family or friends. I still hold a few individuals in pretty low esteem. That's called being a flawed human. I simply don't clutter my mind with them anymore. Again, a waste of my time and energy; they truly are not worth it. Let them go. Cancer teaches you that karma, or the universe, or whatever force it may be, will take care of everything from here on out. These people already put the energy and futility into the cycle. This applies to us as well. No need to add more. Waste on waste is just more waste. I know. Profound. Let the universe handle it. You take care of you. Be the best you. That's the most powerful revenge out there. Much to my surprise, the minute I intentionally chose to let all of that garbage flush down the toilet, my mind cleared to focus on everyone who truly matters and opened real estate for me to exert energies on the betterment and lifting up of myself and others. It allowed me to fill my heart, and soul, full of love. Tossing love and well-wishes out into the universe is like releasing dandelions in the wind. It's easy. They spread in the breeze. They plant themselves elsewhere. They form roots. They grow. It just takes someone pulling the dandelion out of the ground. I needed to be pulled; my roots were firmly set before all this. I've said it before, but it warrants restating. I was not honoring that true warrior spirit. Being completely satiated with love leaves no vacancy for hatred or vengeance. There were other, more relevant, more positive, and more productive battles to fight. And that, my friends, is time and energy well spent.

Hi Kaye,

Sending you love, well-wishes, and happy thoughts! I wanted to send you a note to let you know that you are in my thoughts and prayers.

Keep kicking ass!

Love,

K.R.

Hey friend!

Some days . . . the supply of available swear words is insufficient to meet the demands. WTF? Hang in there! Hope this puts a smile on your face. Please know you're in my prayers every day. You got this!

Love,

E.M.

Chapter 8: Warriors Never Battle Alone

$$\left\{ \begin{array}{c} \textit{Manifest plainness, embrace simplicity,} \\ \textit{reduce selfishness, have few desires.} \\ \textit{~Lao Tzu~} \end{array} \right\}$$

Cancer takes its toll on EVERY. ONE. EV-ER-Y-ONE.

I spend a good deal of windshield time, bonding with my car and Audible books, for my job. I enjoy the open road, meeting and collaborating with brilliant and dedicated individuals, and discovering new locations. It's a sense of mild adventure in a work setting that leads to further exploration during non-work time.

During one of the most recent drives around the state, I came across a billboard that caught my eye. Granted, I was speeding along the interstate, so I had to make sure I paid closer attention on my return trip. I could tell it was for a medical facility that displayed a man, maybe in his thirties, curled up with a young boy on a sofa. The young boy was donning a superhero cape and didn't look well. The caption on the billboard read, "Every sidekick needs a superhero." Truth. I'm just the sidekick in all of this. Dave is my hero. My children and grands are my heroes. Past survivors are my heroes. Caretakers are my true heroes. Nurses, doctors, and medical experts and researchers are my heroes. They're the ones getting survivors back up and moving onward not only to surviving but also to thriving. They're the ones ensuring that some day, one day, we find a cure. I don't want to be a survivor, a two-time survivor, a three-time survivor. I want to be much more: I plan to *thrive*. This first time. I aim to be well. I aim to be whole. I aim to give back. I aim to live a healthy, long, and simple life with the people I love the most. If we each take an honest, long look at our wrestling matches with whiplash and adversity, we are only able to fulfill our sidekick duties because of our superheroes along this entire journey. Sir Isaac Newton is credited with saying, "If I have seen further than others, it is by standing upon the shoulders of giants." Those giants are our superheroes. Just as we embrace the mythology of Amazon warriors and the heroes that have emerged from legends passed down, embrace your heroes. They're everywhere, but sometimes you have to seek them out. No matter how they come into your life, they come into your life for a reason. They are your comrades in battle. But you probably won't see them donning capes.

I can't imagine the turmoil my mom might have experienced during all of this. We really didn't talk about it much, but I'm sure she suffered in silence with many uncertainties. As a parent, watching our children during times of crisis is crushing. I'm not talking about the time I got all worked up about a grade I thought my child didn't deserve. It wasn't the tirade I went on about playing time. It wasn't the comforting sobs at their bedsides when a friend excluded them. Nope, none of that. Helplessness as a parent comes rushing back when I recall two moments of crippling crisis, when my abilities and efforts as a parent were completely useless.

In the summer of 2009, shortly following his high school graduation, our son, Jordan, enlisted in the US Army and left for Basic Training. A self-admitted helicopter mom, it was incredibly unsettling that our youngest child was not only fleeing the nest, but also flying thousands of miles away to get trampled and beaten down physically, mentally, and emotionally. That's Basic Training, I was informed. We spent our summer looking forward to the Sunday night calls, as that was the only correspondence we were allowed to have besides snail mail letters, which I wrote every single day. On July 9, 2009, I spent a glorious summer day, free of humidity and mosquitoes, at a local farmers market, picking up a beautiful bounty of fresh, healthy, locally-grown produce to bring home to create something decadent. I was going into full-on food prep mode with this cornucopia. Then, the call came. It was one of Jordan's friend's mother.

"Kaye? This is Mike's mom. Is now a good time to talk?" I could tell by the cracks in her voice this wasn't going to be good.

"I'm afraid I have some bad news. There was an accident yesterday." Silence. Sniffling.

"She didn't make it." There it was again—deer in headlights.

It was a fairly new relationship and one we knew very little about, but at that time, Jordan was seeing a young lady he had met at school. As the nosy mom, I'm sure there were incredibly viable reasons I was kept out of the "relationship memo" loop. We really hadn't gotten to know her very well yet, but she had planned to come with us to watch his graduation from Basic Training later in the month. Now, she was gone.

This was on a Tuesday. We were not going to talk to Jordan until Sunday. That was hard enough. It was that moment, once I had numbly thanked the caller and began putting the farmers market goodies in their respective places, I realized I was completely helpless. There would be no farmers market creations today. *How would I tell him? What would I say? How would he react? What if despair, and all the fatigue that Basic thrusts upon cadets, causes him to do something drastic? What if he quits? What if? What if? What if?* We clearly had never dealt with an event like this before in our lives as a family. I did not know what to do. I was so inadequate at this. I called the Red Cross, his ROTC office, I even talked to the chaplain assigned to his post. I was lost. I could not wait until Sunday, but Sunday it was. I spent the remaining five days in a fog. I cried every day. I sought answers to get Jordan on the phone sooner but to no avail. Crushed and paralyzed, we made it to Sunday, and the inevitable phone call and unconsolable hysteria ensued. First, it was my sobs, then it was his. For another few weeks until graduation, we were frozen with helplessness. I worried about his welfare, his mental state, his ability to cope, the support he would or wouldn't receive, and his drive to rise above it until he could get home. Dave and I attended her funeral service and awkwardly introduced ourselves to her mother. Apparently, she had been left out of the "need-to-know" mom loop, too, but we sent regards from Jordan, who could not leave Basic Training to attend. When he arrived home later that month, I rode with him to her grave site so he could say goodbye on his own terms. Somehow, time would heal as it always does. It just didn't seem like it at the moment. Jordan grew stronger. He increased his desire to serve. He met his wonderful wife, Samantha, in ROTC training. For all of this, I am grateful. That said, it was the first time I couldn't do a single thing for my own child. I had nothing to offer to help my own son. Helpless. Hopeless. Worthless. Even an Amazon warrior feels this way. No matter how strong we are, there are simply moments in life that bring us to our knees.

In the spring of 2016, our daughter, Ashley, a young mother of two, discovered she had a brain tumor. There had been some ongoing, albeit subtle, warning signs for years, but she attributed them to stress, overdoing it on the basketball court, or sleeping on a wonky pillow. We had never really considered something as serious as a tumor as the cause of these recurring symptoms, for Pete's sake! This was compounded by a cruel, ruthless divorce and all of the evil and unsettling feelings that accompanied it. But the divorce, as awful as it was, was completely eclipsed by this. There was no sleep. There was no concentration on anything else. There was that damn deer-in-the-headlights feeling again. Helpless. Hopeless. Dumbfounded. Damnit! I WebMD'd everything I possibly could about brain tumors. Again, I cried almost every day. I thought about her precious children nonstop. And often, at the most inopportune times. I worried about the three of them constantly. I sought guidance. I again relied heavily on friends. I can say we visualized, and petitioned, nothing but a positive outcome. I meditated endlessly, at all hours, about the removal of the tumor and her health returning to normal as soon as possible. We had all agreed that we would hope for the best and prepare for the worst. And, with all my might, I put on my determined warrior princess face and shielded myself with upbeat attitude armor so she couldn't see how badly I was shattering into a million pieces on the inside. And friends, I kid you not, that is *exactly* how I got my cancer. I'm convinced. *I asked for it.* Repeatedly and without abandon, during every single one of my contemplations, I pleaded that if anyone in our family had to go through cancer, please, please, please—it needed to be me. Maybe it's part of that warrior self-sacrificing mentality, but it's honestly how I felt. Not my kids. Not my mom. Not my grands. Not my siblings. Not my family. Not my friends who were (and still are) family. Not my husband. ME. Throughout this book, I write about my belief in karma and the higher power of the universe often. I asked the universe. Turns out, her tumor was benign and almost completely removed. She had been through a hellish, but successful, nine-hour surgery. She was relentless in her recovery, but it took time. Again, helplessness reared its ugly head, and we needed to rely on each other and time to survive, heal, and eventually, thrive.

I've been known to get my way quite frequently throughout my adult life, but this was beyond any logical explanation. Much like the Amazon warrior, Hippolyta, I wielded a propensity for overpowering abilities in persuasion. Be careful what you ask for.

"You're welcome," smirked the universe.

Both of these instances brought me back to what my mom might have experienced during my battle with cancer. I'm not sure. She did not share her fears with me. She called and checked in frequently for updates. She knew I had Dave with me. I can only rely on my own experiences as a mother to even remotely relate to what she must have felt. Every parent handles their children's turmoils differently. You have your way, I have mine. This cancer journey gave me pause to consider how much, or how little, we as parents can actually do to help our kids through the muck.

Then, there's Dave, my husband and, in complete disregard of being cliché, my best friend for over thirty-five years. We often get a lighthearted chuckle at how young couples announce their engagements on social media about marrying their "best friends." It's so sweet. Sorry not sorry, it strikes me as somewhat amusing. Hear me out. It's incredible and powerful when we meet that "certain someone" with whom we instantly connect. The one with whom we adventure. The one with whom we laugh until snot spews from our noses. The one with whom we cry when our child has an uncontrollable cough or when a pet crosses over the rainbow bridge. The one with whom we compete—over what? Oh, I'm not quite sure, but we sure do love to compete. The one we love with every fiber of our being—on the days of nonexistent romance, the days of big dreaming and plan making, the days of swearing, the days of eye rolls, the days of immeasurable joy, and the days of shattering pain. That is cool! Here's my point. Dave and I knew we'd be together, probably forever, because, truth be told, we're both kind of "interesting" to live with. We started out getting each others' names messed up. I thought he said his name was Henri, and he thought my name was Kayla. It stuck. We began our journey together struggling to make ends meet and deciding which bill could be sacrificed to pay another each month. We started out with a family. We started out with dreams and goals, both individual and shared, and we allowed each other to go after those individual goals while working diligently on the shared ones. We agreed that when our children were young, Dave would be the worker bee, building his coaching career, and I would be primarily responsible for our children's activities. This was mutual, and this worked. A shift in this partnership, career-supporting activity happened when both of our eaglets flew the nest. My career was more clearly in focus, and he took on more responsibility with our home—inside and out. We have a great life, and it's something neither of us are willing to let go. We've compromised, sacrificed, celebrated, and depended heavily on each other in times of need. There's so much remaining for us to do, and as Jon Bon Jovi *(man, I love Bon Jovi!)* so eloquently rocked out, "We're halfway there . . . " So yes, Dave— or Henri as most people know him—is my best friend, for better or worse, in sickness and in health. This was definitely one of those "in sickness" moments people promise but sometimes forget.

The thing is, the longer you spend with "the one," the more creative and patient and innovative you become in a partnership. Not everything is puppy dogs and unicorn glitter farts. You can't wake up one day and suddenly decide you're unhappy and bail. It takes work. It takes communication. It takes revisiting goals. It takes time. With each other. Through honest, and sometimes excruciating, conversations. Nobody likes doing any of that, but if it's worth fighting for, it's worth the brawl . . . and the emotional bruising. It was this journey with cancer and the culmination of other life events that brought Dave and I to the conclusion that once you have single-handedly carried each other through fire ant hills, piles of feces, and every firestorm that has come your way, either individually or as a couple, you can call each other your best friend. In true warrior princess fashion, best friends band together through the dirty, messy, sticky, hairy, unsexy, and downright gross and maddening battles of life, and cancer is, without a doubt, all of those things combined and magnified . . . plus rabid fire ants up your pant leg. In peanut butter.

Dave and I often share with people how we've seen each other at our best and at our worst. Well honey, you ain't seen nothing until you face cancer. See, a cancer diagnosis doesn't impact just the one carrying around the deadly killer; it impacts everyone within reach. It reminds me of an atomic bomb—you've got the center of contact (where I was lucky enough to be positioned), and then you have the circumference of ripples that demolishes anything in its path as collateral damage. That's what I see for caretakers and loved ones sustaining those battling cancer. For well over a year's time, Dave didn't know what to say, what to do, what to cook, what not to cook, where to touch, what to avoid, where the tissue box was again . . . and the list goes on. And yes, I am keenly aware that countless others deal with a diagnosis and subsequent treatments for much longer with less than a cheery and promising prognosis. He had to deal with me losing memories, my keys, my dinner, my physical body, and my mind. Deer in the headlights. Again. Damn deer.

Here's where I get super vulnerable and, quite honestly, selfish. I thought that once I was diagnosed, there would be a circling of wagons and the love and support would shower in, especially by those closest to me. I've seen it and have been part of it when others went through similar situations. Funny thing is, some of my most adamant and committed supporters came from the farthest corners of my life circles, both relationally and geographically. Don't get me wrong. I'm sure our mail carrier had had enough of the constant packages, cards, and loads of generosity from dozens of people. People who cared. We had a profusion of visitors, even more lasagna and casseroles (comfort food upholds its moniker for a reason, people!), and endless calls, texts, social media outreach, and just plain care. For all of those actions of kindness and well-wishes, I will never feel adequate enough with my thanks and appreciation. It also pains me to think of those I shared waiting rooms with, who had no one. They were in this all alone. It still breaks my heart, and strains my heart, to think of how we can better ensure that no one goes this road alone without other warriors beside them for strength.

I didn't see that vast outreach from a few people I thought were closest to me. I'm not sure why. Maybe I shouldn't have expected it. I don't know. *Had I done something to them at some point that they pretty much ignored that I was going through this horrendous challenge? Was it fear? Was it intolerance? Did they avoid asking how I was so they didn't have to listen to lovely small talk about constipation, brutal scars and battles burns, and complete, unadulterated whining?* I don't have a clue. It remains a mystery to me, but nothing I dwell on much because like the diagnosis and treatment itself, everyone deals with adversity in incredibly unique ways . . . and sometimes those ways end up unintentionally hurting others. I know I am guilty of this. It might actually be a combination of all these things. Heaven knows, I'm no saint, nor have I ever claimed to be one. Something prevented them from reaching out, and we can leave it at that. Dwelling on "Why me?" or "Why not me?" never resulted in me getting anything I yearned for, really. So I stopped. It's pointless. I think sometimes, as caretakers or supporters, we just don't know what to do or what to say. I could certainly identify. I understood this. All I know is that it hurt at the time. A lot. (Okay, the violins-warrior rant is over.)

When I go on one of my far too many visits to a doctor's office—oncology, radiation oncology, plastic surgery, lab (they love me in the lab—I win an achievement award for having "wicked awesome" veins, apparently)—I pass the time observing. I love watching people. I scan the room, see who's there, notice age, gender, ethnicity. I will admit I die a little bit inside every time I see children. No bones about it, kids should *never* have to experience cancer. Ever. I notice how many patients are accompanied by someone else. I also notice the ones flying solo. During a recent visit, I noticed a familiar-faced woman, maybe in her sixties or early seventies, I had encountered several times before. She's there. Every time. All alone. As if sitting in an oncology waiting area didn't already induce melancholy, her solitude struck a sorrowful chord in me. This time I was alone—one of the very few times I was—so I struck up a conversation with her. Her husband had recently passed away. They had owned and operated a little dairy farm about an hour from the medical facility out in the bluffed countryside, and her adult children were traveling hundreds of miles to come help her care for the farm and all the innumerable responsibilities that came with maintaining it. They had started talking about selling the farm. It was just too much for her to manage on her own, ya know. They were packing up the treasures she and her husband had accumulated over forty-five years of marriage into cardboard boxes labeled with a black Sharpie®. Her life was being boxed up back at the farm. In here, her life was now in question. She was heartbroken. I could sense it in her words.

Her family had "important" things to do, after all, so she had a neighbor drop her off and pick her up here. She so very calmly lamented losing everything as she smiled meekly. I'm a crier by nature. Where's a damn tissue when you need one? We made small talk about our families, diagnoses, and subsequent treatment plans, and eventually, she made her way in to see the doctor. I was grateful that this time I had a delay in my appointment so I could pull myself together. I never did see her in the waiting room again.

They say people come into our lives for a reason. This was no exception. She was sent to me to help me realize how insanely fortunate I was to have the people I had in my corner. It's amazing how epiphanies can show up in the most peculiar places and at unexpected moments. I was at this one, single, solitary appointment by myself, and I just about lost my mind. Good grief! She helped me abruptly dispel any "poor me" choruses I thought I needed about people not reaching out. Plenty did. Today, even more continue to do so. *You have an army, warrior princess. She is a lone soldier. Stop it, self.*

You know, friends, any time we're smacked in the head with adversity, and that includes being overlooked, passed by, or ignored, we have two choices: Become bitter or become better. Again, the words of Josh Shipp. When things like this happen, it's super easy to fall into bitterness. In all honesty, I did for a while. I want to believe it's an element of human nature. I spent moments mulling over people's reasonings behind their inactions. I swooped into melancholy on those rare occasions when I went to appointments alone. Even though I had destined myself to stay away from self pity, I do recall one or two times when I sent myself a "no plus one" invite to my own, ridiculous pity party. For a brief interlude, the pity made me angrier. And let me tell you, anger kills. It might be a swift, head-on collision. It may be a slow and festering boil, but anger can kill. I made a harrowing transition to stop the *bitter* right there. Right then. I chose *better* over *bitter*. Don't let *bitter* ever find its way to you. No more pity parties.

This kismet-filled encounter with my "friend in cancer" helped shaped my priorities; I've learned to focus only on the good. It has helped with my vision—the ability to see how others feel. Do everything I can in my power not only to give back, but somehow pay it forward. Focus on finding a way to support those affected by cancer through regional support groups, something acutely missing from our little neck of the woods. When we devote our time to building each other up, there's no space for bitterness, jealousy, and knocking each other down. Think about it. The Amazons did it all the time. They trained their up-and-coming protégés in horseback riding, sword wielding, and battle strategy. By lifting each other up, their entire community was stronger. I remember thinking that no matter how bad things seemed for me during this journey (and it's not completed yet, by any means), someone else's is far worse. An open mind will always open the heart.

Pity party over. It ain't just about me. Point taken.

Henri
Ain't it great; Ain't it fine
To have a love—someone—that others can't find
Ain't it wonderful to know all we ever need is just the two of us
She and I
~David Loggins~

I was going to entitle this section, "Dave," because you, dear reader, might not know that he is Henri to everyone in our town, including the kids who know him as "Coach Henri." My partner in crime. When I say no one does this alone, I'm not kidding. There's this boy I met way back when, donning a red flannel fishing shirt and drinking Mountain Dew. He asked me to dance. He had been at an ice fishing contest all day (it's what we do in Wisconsin to embrace January). I was on my annual "Girls Only, Anti-Male Weekend," with big AquaNet hair and leg warmers to boot. We failed awkwardly on this first encounter. He got my name wrong. I got his name wrong. We danced. We dated. I never participated in G.O.A.M. Weekend again. The rest is a beautiful history of love, adventure, friendship, and true and reciprocal admiration.

Far too often, much of the cancer journey is focused on the patient, the survivor. While it's important to remember this, we can't ignore how we got where we are. Our superheroes. There are scores of literature and support resources for survivors. The jury is still out on substantial support resources for caretakers, the wonderful people who survivors lean on most for support. It's one thing to focus on yourself when you're attempting to kick a killer in the ass; it's quite another to recognize and honor those who ride beside you during the whole battle.

This is Henri's (Dave, to those meeting him for the first time) story:

It was Friday, January 6. I was processing the fall harvest of venison at Jerry's with the guys. It's something we typically did at the beginning of each year to have enough ground, steaks, hot dogs, bologna, etc. from our fall harvest for the next year. I knew you were at your appointment, but it didn't distract from enjoying some laughter with the guys. I became worried when I saw it was you on my caller ID, wondering what the news might be. It didn't take long to feel sick to my stomach. Butterflies turned to bad cheese in my gut. I felt like a complete heel for not being there for the biopsy. You reassured me before you left. You said it would be no big deal—just another negative, false alarm, and you would meet me at home when I was done. We would have a Friday night fish fry, like any other typical end-of-the-work-week Friday night. I immediately had to leave what I was doing to be home when you got there. I heard you sob. I heard you swear. I heard your pain in your words. I couldn't do a single thing to make you feel better. You sounded angry, but I know you well enough to know this is how you get when you're scared. I briefly explained things to the guys, and they guaranteed they would take care of everything, then they sent me home. I knew I couldn't take back not being there with you initially; I was paralyzed. I oddly felt like a failure as a husband. I couldn't do anything to calm your fears. All I could think of was, *Why? Why did this happen?* Almost instantly, my mind went to what our future was going to look like. Everything we had planned, our upcoming travel adventures, retirement dreams, building projects . . . all in question. It was the most frightened I've ever been in my life. Nothing, I mean nothing, prepared me for this.

I made it my mission to be at every appointment I could from there on out. I needed to get the thousands of questions I had in my brain answered: *What were the next steps? What was the process we had to complete to survive? What could I do?* I was consumed with worry about what every test result would show, and there were a lot of tests. The medical terminology was a whole new world for me. I had never had much exposure to any of these terms, but you read and read and read to learn, and that's what we did. Our ordinary Friday nights, or any other nights for that matter, turned into days and nights of learning, reading, commiserating, planning, crying, and the big positive of all this time at home, dog cuddling. The stark contrast between hearing about someone going through cancer and actually experiencing it firsthand became obvious to me. Every appointment was filled with the suspense of not knowing what to expect or what to do. This whole thing was unknown, and for this, I should be grateful. We had never experienced anything like this before. My father had battled cancer, but he and my mother dealt with it in their own way and did not share a whole lot of detail or specifics. They handled it together, and my brother and I helped where we were needed. But this was new. We were the ones on the front lines now. Answers weren't coming fast enough. I found myself growing impatient with the process and with all the delays, the extra biopsies, the CT scans, the surgical consult, the treatment plan appointment, and on and on. The wheels on this bus weren't moving fast enough for me; I wanted to start taking action right away. Everything I did know about cancer, which was pretty limited up to that point, screamed early detection, early detection, early detection, and there we were, spending six weeks to two months on tests. In my head, your life depended on it. We needed to move. Right then and there.

Enter helplessness. I knew we had a serious issue in front of us, and we had to rely on everyone besides ourselves to find a solution. We've always been ones who tackle problems together. We do what needs to be done, we get results. Together. But we had to wait. There was only so much we could do independently. This was new for us. We had to rely on others. And think positively. And stay focused on the outcomes we wanted. And not freak out every single minute of every single day.

So, we finally reached a point where we had a plan. After spending my entire career coaching and mentoring student athletes, my brain only functioned one way. I needed to process all of this like a game plan: Goals. Steps. Monitoring. Action plans. Results. Evaluate. Repeat. That's how I'm wired. It's the only way I could make something that made no sense at all into something we could unravel. We had some deep, distressing decisions to make. We had to weigh lumpectomy versus mastectomy, and up until this point, I never really had any reason to truly understand either of them. Once I wrapped my head around the definitions and implications of each, coupled with a rudimentary understanding of the diagnosis, we thought we had reached a relatively easy option . . . until we sat in the surgical consult and were forced to sign on the dotted line. Literally. You repeatedly expressed your concerns for *me* losing *your* breasts. My feelings about losing something physical that quite frankly, we both enjoyed. We've been together for a long, long time. I just needed you. To live. To survive. To come back to me with your typical fire and warrior mentality. I wanted you back. Everything else was cosmetic. End of discussion.

Surgery day. We arrived early for check-in. It was still black as night in the wee hours of the morning. It would be a long day.

We both knew that. You, of course, had everything packed and organized for your stay in recovery. The seventy-five minute drive to the hospital seemed so short because the time had finally come. We were there. We were ready. This was it. We had done all the homework. We had prepared meals, paid the bills, cleaned the house, fed the dog, all in preparation for a return to focus entirely on healing. This was the next step on the road to survival, to getting you back to where we both needed you to be. We were acutely aware that nothing would be the same after that day. Checking in and being in the pre-op room left me in a state of renewed suspense, not really knowing what the day would entail. It hurt to leave you alone in the pre-op room. We do everything together—the good, the not-so-awesome, the sometimes ugly, and now I was leaving you all alone. I went to the waiting room, and there I sat. Numb.

I drank my weight in coffee that day. This obviously led to a lot of alone time in the restroom, partially from coffee consumption but mostly to pull myself together. I'm not ashamed to say how scared I was. The unknowns take their time flying through your brain when you're waiting for someone you love to come out of surgery. My mind was consumed with how you were doing and how surgery was progressing. Even though your mom and sister were there with me the whole time, my attempts at small talk and being present were grand levels of failure. I was incredibly distracted. I couldn't hold a conversation for any length of time. I was with you. I wanted you out of there. I found myself checking the waiting room monitor at least a thousand times—you know, the one that had your patient number on it, displaying which part of the surgical process you were in. Five hours, and even more coffee later, you were sent to recovery. Instead of getting to see you right away, I met with your surgeons. Alone. Remember? We do everything together. I was uneasy. The suspense and not knowing led me to do something I normally would never do. I could not eat. Anyone who knows me knows how much I like to keep my energy levels up and how much I love a good meal. Nothing was appetizing that day. I couldn't eat a thing. The only time I have ever gotten sick was when I didn't eat, yet that day was different. My mind was nowhere near thoughts of food. I was already sick. Not sick in my stomach but sick in my heart. Then, the surgeons came out. Talking to them left me with an initial sigh of relief. The surgery had gone exceptionally well. The first leg of the journey had been successful. You were in recovery. That in itself was a whole new issue.

For whatever reason, you were not coming out of anesthesia very quickly. It took you longer than normal to wake up. During what seemed like another eternity of wait time, I updated everyone about your status. I busied myself with texts and social media updates. It was at this point I once again needed to separate myself from your sister and mom so I could pull myself together and absorb all the return messages of well-wishes we had received. I was overwhelmed with emotion by the barrage of support from afar. I was also somewhat concerned that I had just told everyone that you were doing well, but yet you were taking your own sweet time in la-la land. It was particularly emotional for me to talk to my mom and brother on the phone. They knew what I was going through, and talking to them about you brought my heart to my throat. Again. It's quite the challenge trying to talk on your cell while not getting electrocuted by your own tears. I thought I had cried myself out. That was silly. I would quickly learn that there would be many more tears throughout this entire process. And that was okay.

It was a massive relief when you finally came to. Why you stayed under so long, no one seems to know. Everyone reacts to anesthesia differently, we were told. Knowing you would be staying the night following your surgery was another step toward finding some solace. Once I gathered myself together and contemplated the next steps in our journey, I knew my next role would be that of nurse and caretaker with all that a bilateral mastectomy entailed. As a coach and athletic director for over thirty years, I had seen and administered aid to more than my share of injuries and wounds. This would be unlike any of those experiences. It was such a welcome sight seeing you come out of surgery, even though you were hopped up on some pretty powerful and gnarly surgery drugs! I should have recorded some of the things you said, but that's for another time. Another book. It was just good to have you back.

When I brought you home, I knew the next few weeks were crucial in your healing process. I won't lie; surgical drain care takes a lot of precision, and quite honestly, while highly beneficial in reducing any risk of infection, they're gross. We agreed to do whatever we needed to make certain they could be removed as soon as possible. I needed to handle this procedure accurately to expedite the healing process and get them gone. I give nurses an enthusiastic standing ovation for what they do to ensure patient safety and forward movement in healing! They walked me through every step of training, and while I was uneasy with the task, I knew we needed to do it. Next came sleep. Lots of it was required. For someone who has resisted napping for as long as I've known you, you spent a lot of time sleeping. Those first days, you were not going to be alone. Even though our home had become a revolving door of visitors, which was nice, I didn't want you to compromise your recovery. I never realized I could enjoy binge-watching mindless TV as much as I did during those first few weeks of recovery. I'll be honest, I did enjoy the pans of lasagna or ready-to-eat meal offers from everyone. It took one thing off the caretaker to-do list—dinner. And, it was always delicious, always comforting, and always appreciated. My love of food had returned.

St. Patrick's Day of 2017 was one I will always remember—not with much fondness, either. We've always found a way to have fun and celebrate being whatever small percentage of Irish we were. We traditionally spend it in Madison, enjoying high school boys' state basketball games and some green lager. That year would be entirely different. We had a follow-up surgical consult, and it turned out that your tumor was much larger and more aggressive than we had initially thought. We went from an uncompromisingly optimistic Stage II to a lot less confident Stage III. Before this, radiation was a question mark in your treatment course, and now it was an undeniable certainty. We were both quite stunned, and I remember we went to grab some lunch, but neither of us had much of an appetite. We just wanted to go home. Our safe place. Cuddle the dog. No festivities. No jubilation. No green beer.

With the first phase of this journey behind us and you well on your way to healing, the next punch in the face came in the form of chemo treatments. Again, you would not do this alone. Eight treatments, eight trips every other week to the hospital. I would be there. And once again, the questions. *How sick would you get from the treatments? Would you be able to have any type of normalcy in your daily activities? Would the poisons be enough to kill the cancer? What else would it kill?* The first round of treatments lasted only forty-five minutes a pop. We could usually grab some groceries or some lunch before heading home. The side effects of chemo were fairly predictable. What you would experience during the first treatment, you would likely experience during the remaining treatments, only with increased intensity and severity as we got closer to the last one. What a two weeks. We had grown accustomed to you having ridiculous amounts of energy during the two days following your treatments. You called them "Steroid Saturdays and Sundays." Funny girl. This also meant you were wide awake at one o'clock in the morning, doing laundry or shuffling around on your laptop, sending out work emails. I'm sure your colleagues got a kick out of those. Sometimes, I would awaken, and we would just talk. Sometimes we'd cry. It was actually nice. We could shut out the entire world and just be real for a few hours before putting the armor back on. Then you'd sleep, sometimes fifteen to eighteen hours a day at the beginning. The second week of each treatment cycle brought an odd sense of normalcy. You could work. You would come home and sleep right away, but you could function. It was tough watching you fight colds and worry about infections throughout the whole chemo process. You never had much of anything more than a sniffle prior to this, and it was tough not seeing you at your strongest, like normal.

The second round of treatments took much longer—three

hours this time. We would sit in a plain, almond-colored room with inspirational quotes painted on the walls like, "Never, ever give up," "Don't go there until you get there," and "Believe in the power of a positive attitude." All helpful. We had gotten to know these walls all too well. Each second round treatment put you to sleep the whole time, something completely new to me—you don't like naps. A guy can only do so many crossword puzzles or word finds. We had talked about the family room remodel, and we had talked about laying a tile floor. I had some background knowledge on the "how to," but I found myself hanging out on YouTube, reviewing the skills needed for laying plank porcelain tiles for our new den floor during your treatment naps. I also occupied my time with something called "Ice Junkies," a group on social media that totally gets into all types of in-season fishing in informative, and somewhat comedic, fashion. It kept my mind focused on what was pleasant and productive and not on how I desperately wanted you to wake up so we could just go home. There would be no stop for groceries or lunch following these treatments. We'd return home so you could rest and allow the poison to kick in and do its thing.

I knew how much you wanted to do, and the reality of it was you couldn't. That was hard to watch. We tried camping, something you love. Any type of excursion was limited by your level of fatigue and lowered immune system. We quickly learned after the first couple of treatments what our life would be like for the next sixteen weeks. When they tell you it's a roller coaster ride, they're not lying. We knew what each day of the two-week cycle would be like. A large percentage of those days were not pleasant, to say the least, and we learned to just deal with it, knowing that you were one step closer. In my incessant attempts to keep things positive, we developed a countdown, starting with eight. You were neither impressed nor did you find any positivity in it when I came up with the idea. You came around when one of your nurses mentioned the countdown process and how it could help. Then it was okay. Good to know you never lost your stubborn warrior princess mentality through all of this.

The last chemo was indeed special for a few reasons. Throughout the whole chemo process, we were fortunate enough to have our daughter, Ashley, visit with her two children for an instant pick-me-up. They always brought laughter, curiosity, and tremendous light and life into our home when we needed it the most. They asked questions, and we were honest with them. B.D. even asked if he could have your wigs when you were done with them. What a kid! The last chemo treatment was July 6. Our son, Jordan, happened to be home on leave from his assignment in the US Army, and he insisted on attending your last treatment. We hadn't seen him or his wife, Sam, and our grandson, K.J., in months. During the last of the three-hour-nap treatments, you fell asleep right away. Once you were out, Jordan and I decided we needed to commemorate the completion and closure of this leg of the mission. As you finished up the last of the treatment, he brought in a chocolate cake with chocolate frosting (your favorite) with "No More Chemo" written in, of course, chocolate icing. We had bright smiley balloons and joined the nurses in singing and blowing bubbles in celebration. No bells to ring. Not yet. That would come after the last leg—radiation. Smiles all around, another sigh of relief. From there, we waited and watched as the poison ran its course and did what it needed to do to keep you alive. It's funny because once we were done with this step, we thought we were completely done. We never took into account that it would take several more months for you to return to any sense of normalcy in your routine. Neither of us were patient, or primed, for that delay in jumping back into life as we knew it again. Another pause.

There was another small surgery between chemo and radiation. The waiting time in between was nerve-racking. It was reassuring to see you slowly regain some strength and stamina again after chemo, only to know there was another step in all this. A nice little incline on the roller coaster ride, only to get knocked down again. We were finally able to do some of the things we enjoyed doing together so much like fishing, travel, some camping. That period was short-lived with the impending radiation. We were not prepared for what radiation had in store. We were under the impression that we had the most challenging procedures behind us. You went to the treatments on your own because they were only twenty minutes long, and you typically went to work when you were done. It was around Halloween. With two weeks remaining in your radiation treatments, I had to witness a meltdown like no other . . . and we had been through some pretty heady meltdowns during all of this. At that point, I realized how important it was for me to take on a more active role in these last couple of weeks because of the intense pain you were experiencing because of the burning and the immense emotional and physical toll it was taking. I learned that sometimes you don't have to have answers; you just need to be present. Neither of us realized how severe the burns would be and how much care they would require to heal once the process was complete. That's when I got to wear my "nurse hat" again. Sometimes you just don't know what you need to do until you're smack dab in the middle of doing it.

No one really coaches caretakers when you experience a cancer journey with someone you love. "Normal" was completely blown out of the water and something we rarely experienced during 2017. Some of the greatest challenges for me were never knowing how much energy you'd have, what your appetite would be like, what emotions would rear their ugly heads. *Would you be calm today? Would you combust into tears today? What activities could we do? What activities should we not do? Should I stay? Should I give you some space?* Never knowing. Pretty much anything. I never knew. Every day was a mystery for me. I recall waking each morning, wishing I had answers when in reality, I had none. Focus was a challenge for me. I knew I had work to do; I had clients who relied on me. Yet, in the back of my head, I was always thinking about you, my better half. (I know you will argue this designation with me.) I just wasn't good at tuning any of this out.

One of the most beneficial, but difficult, decisions we made was to go ahead with the family room remodel. I was able to keep busy and keep my mind on construction-related topics while never leaving you alone. I was busy laying tiles; you helped when you could. It was refreshing to get activity in when you were feeling up to it, even though there were clearly times you overdid it. Then, there was my sanctuary—the woods. When I knew you were resting and wanted me out of the house, I ran away—literally—to my safe haven. I was able to connect with nature, run my chainsaw, get some exercise, and most importantly, enjoy one of my passions to clear my head. I texted you to see how you were doing, and I knew that if need be, I was only minutes away. I wonder how many other caretakers out there have some type of positive outlet. We all need to take care of ourselves, and if we go down, so does our ability to care for our loved ones. You realized that and sent me on my way to play Paul Bunyan in the woods. For that, I am grateful.

Another blessing was reaching out to friends and acquaintances who had either traveled this road before us or were traveling it parallel to us. There's definitely power in commiseration and support, especially when pizza is involved. It's at this point when you realize you're not alone. There's always someone wishing you well. Connection to each other was such an integral component of getting back on our feet. We were in this together. We felt each other's pain. We, at times, got so caught up in the process that we forgot about how much fun we liked to have together. That's why keeping our plans for Cancun (made the previous year) was an absolute priority for us. It was the unintended therapy we needed to fully grasp what this year would throw our way. We also started viewing adventure through new lenses. We had planned a road trip to return Jordan's car to his station in El Paso, Texas. We initially had thought about a two-day trip since the drive was over twenty-two hours long. In a moment of reclaimed strength (or stupidity), you suggested an all-nighter. We were originally going to split driving duties, and I don't know how it came to be, but I was determined to drive the whole route, with you on navigation duty the whole way, with a dogged alertness I never knew I possessed. Cancer can do that to you, too! It puts things in perspective. If you could go through all these treatments, I could stay awake and drive the whole trip. You remained as alert as you could and stayed with me, pointing out all our exits and turns along the way. We make such a great team!

I don't face fear easily or publicly. I like to face it on my own and move forward. I'm not one to make conversation about something that could be interpreted as weakness. Let me tell you—cancer exposes fear after fear after fear, and we had no choice but to talk about them. One of my biggest fears was waiting for test results. *What would pathology say? What would the blood work indicate? Would there be any surprises with a CT or bone scan?* Over and over again. It all felt like a record on repeat in my mind. Like most everything with cancer, those St. Patrick's Day revelations just plastered on a whole new layer of questions and fear.

Failure is another thing I don't readily accept. My first failure was not being there at the onset of this. I assumed that everything would be all right because they always were. Not knowing what all of the new medical terminology meant, not knowing what you could and couldn't do, not knowing where our future was headed. Failure at knowing. I am a firm believer that failure is only failure if you don't learn from it. I learned that when it comes to a battle of this magnitude, you can never be present enough. That is, until you're kicked out of the house for smothering. Then, there's overkill. I just could not, would not, fail you.

I'm often referred to as positively perky. You remind me of this all of the time. I have the ability to see the good in almost everything and everyone. I firmly believe that's a quality worth possessing. With cancer, however, seeing the positive in everything is downright challenging. On one hand, someone you love has just been diagnosed with this beast. On the other hand, when we saw the words "curable" on the oncologist's prognosis, it brightened our hearts. *We're going to cure this. We're going to remove it, poison it, burn it, and kick it to the curb, with any luck, forever.* With all the tests that were run, we had a more thorough understanding of what was going on inside you than most people who had never been diagnosed. Come what may, you summoned the courage to think, "We've got this." And if I ever thought it possible, you and I grew even closer. We've always been kind of like stink on poo, peanut butter and jelly—where one goes, the other follows. Cancer made us cherish our time together and relish the thought of all our adventures to come. We're more immediate with our planning now instead of putting dreams on hold for "down the road." Cancer makes it crystal clear that "down the road" may never come. We've learned to laugh more frequently, love more fervently, and live more intentionally. And for that, I guess in some twisted way, we can thank cancer.

Oh. And for the record, I love your curly hair.

Dave and Kaye,

Not one day goes by when you are not in our thoughts and prayers. The strength and support the two of you share is nothing short of amazing.

We send our love to you and hope that each day is better than the day before. God is watching over you both. We know this because we asked Him to.

Love,

D and S

Kaye,

I just wanted you to know that I have been thinking about and praying for you. I have had this card for quite some time, hence the beat up edges, but I just finally sat down to write what I've been wanting to tell you. I have never met a more inspiring, optimistic, and life-loving person. You truly motivate me to be the best version of myself, each and every day. Your courage and positivity are admirable. I knew there was a reason God brought you into my life, many, many (okay, you're not that old *smiles*) years ago in that sixth-grade classroom.

Keep being you! You touch more lives than you even realize!
S.E.

Chapter 9: Warriors are Human, Too

{ *Look at situations from all angles, and you will become more open.*
~Dalai Lama~ }

DISCLAIMER: *This chapter is not intended to offend anyone, but I understand if it might. Don't let it. Remember, this is my story. My truth. My list of "What Helps" and "What Doesn't." Much of it comes from lessons learned through my inadequacies in trying to support others traversing their own dire circumstances. When it comes to cancer, there is NO one-size-fits-all journey. Learn with me.*

Rainbows and Unicorn Glitter Farts

Nope. Not helpful. My glass is always half full. I'm a self-proclaimed nose-to-the-ground, positive person. I am fully in tune with the research behind the power of positive thinking. If there's a problem, I prefer to devise plans and take stabs at possible solutions. If someone's hurting, I want to ease their pain, although I'm not always successful at that. This may sound odd, but I don't really fall into any singular recognized, organized religious sect. My personal spiritual philosophy is that each organized belief system has a great deal to offer, but each has its limitations and constraints. What they all consistently promote, however, is the notion of "do unto others." A "golden rule" of sorts. I fervently believe in noticing signs around us and harnessing the power of positive thinking and positive visualization. If I had to identify with something, I suppose I could be considered a secular humanist. I believe in humanity. I have immense faith. I believe. I simply don't name my belief. I believe in meditation, which some people might call prayer. I believe in cleansing an aura and centering on gratitude. I believe in medical advances and the research, science, and technology that accompanies them. That's where I choose to exist fundamentally. The here and now. Facing a fear-filled, questionable reality doesn't always lend itself well to entertaining a unicorn glitter mentality. But maybe Amazon warriors rode unicorns. Who knows?

Let's talk about signs. *What led me to find this little pea? What made me perform a self-exam in the shower that particular morning when I had been so consistently inconsistent for years?* I do believe in signs. I didn't always give them much attention or credence. That's changed. A lot. I'm a Libra, and Libras are notorious for strong intuition and sense of balance. Sad to say, I've pretty much ignored both most of my life. More signs of the mythical genre. Whether you choose to believe or not, these come in the form of astrological lore, and for what it's worth, I've always been strangely captivated by them. My Western zodiac tells me I'm the intuitive, overprotective, big-picture, grudge-holding scales of justice Libra. Sounds about right. My Celtic zodiac sign is the butterfly, which means I'm always open to social wandering; I do love people watching as well as meet and greets! Such dreamers butterflies are! They, like me, tend to possess a childlike wonder and inquisitiveness. All true. According to Native American symbolism, I belong to the falcon totem, which indicates a propensity for judgment, swift action, and persistence. Check, check, and check, for good, bad, or indifferent. My Chinese zodiac, based on the year I was born, is the horse. Perfect! Another strong animal likeness. Those of us born in the year of the horse tend to be the wild child, constantly asking questions. Desire and passions tend to overwhelm us—a potential Achilles' heel. That's where I need my Libra self to pull me back into some semblance of balance again. Ummmm . . . yep. Signs. Whether or not any of this had anything to do with why I chose to randomly self-examine that day during Christmas break, leading to the discovery of the pea that would derail my life for a while, remains to be seen. I do know one thing: I won't be ignoring any signs from here on out. Always trust your gut.

Here's where I become a dichotomy. I am a deeply spiritual and contemplative being. I meditate twice daily, once when I wake and once before sleep. I give thanks for breathing, for getting off pain meds, for the health and love of my family and friends, for making it through an entire day without a nap, for having absurdly curly, unmanageable thick hair once again. I ask for strength to deal with the scars, the pieces and parts that are markedly absent, the hole in my heart for those suffering far worse than I, and for peace for my family and friends' hearts and souls. Being real helps; pretending nothing is wrong and that everything will return to normalish the day you're done with treatment does not. Facades and la-la-land just don't work for me because well, they're not real. They're fantasy, and fantasy is not sustainable. It seems futile to me to aspire to lead some utopian existence. I certainly had the option of becoming the queen of denial about all of this or accepting the ugly reality in front of me and do whatever it took to live. Let's be honest. I never asked for things to return to normal. Things will never be normal again. That's reality. Reality isn't always pretty or welcome, but it's a whole lot more palatable than navigating in a make-believe world. The glamorized glory of battle doesn't always match the devastating reality. This shit's for real.

Hysteria

Going zero to dead the minute you hear the diagnosis is exactly what I did, and apparently, it's not an uncommon reaction. I mentioned the power of social media and connecting with others via virtual spaces when you physically cannot connect. The reverse can also be true. Breast cancer support apps, for the most part, were threads of doom for me. There was a lot of answer-seeking, and I learned a great deal from others about side effects or links to explore when looking for apparel or burn cream. It was not negative, per se; it simply felt sad. I didn't need those toxic thoughts. I know these sites benefit thousands of survivors, and for that, I am thankful. I just wasn't one of them. I found myself getting sucked into others' hyperbolic abysses, and it just wasn't healthy. Don't get me wrong. I still think about recurrence. I worry about little aches and pains. *Will I see my grandchildren grow up? Will I live to retirement? Will Dave and I be able to explore all of the places on our travel bucket list?* I think it's safe to say I think more about my mortality now than ever before. Maybe that's normal when you reach a certain age; maybe it was spurred on by this crapfest chain of events. However, these thoughts don't completely consume my time. There's just so much more to do than ruminate incessantly. I've been guilty of clumping all breast cancer diagnoses into one bucket. In reality, there are no two women (or men) who will have a diagnosis (and subsequent treatment regimen) identical to someone else. There are more than one hundred chemotherapy drugs on the market. Yes, certain ones are designed specifically for breast cancer, which makes generalizations dangerous. That's what I was finding in these online support communities, sadly. They simply didn't work for me.

Around the one-year anniversary of my chemo treatments, former First Lady Barbara Bush passed. News outlets, both mainstream and social media, shared part of the commencement speech she delivered to Wellesley College graduates in 1990. Funny how timely this lovely lady's words were almost thirty years later as I attempted to calm the waters of hysteria and resume my trek to normalish again:

"At the end of your life, you will never regret not having passed one more test, winning one more verdict, or not closing one more deal. You will regret time not spent with a child, a friend, or a parent."

Hysteria. Done.

The Shoulda, Woulda, Coulda Club

Oh my goodness! When you share a cancer diagnosis out loud, people are insanely wonderful! Tater tot casserole and lasagna show up out of nowhere. Lotions, potions, and creams are plentiful. Advice abounds. You get everything from, "Did you know this beet root cures cancer?" to "If it were me, there's no way I'd go through chemo and radiation." It's all well-meaning. I get it. It all comes from a good place. I firmly believe that. It just doesn't help. Without a doubt, it stems from others' desires to lift you up . . . the one actually living the hell of chemo . . . and radiation . . . and all the cutting. They try, but they just haven't experienced it.

"You can use this as motivation." Wait. What?! I can't even express how preposterous this sounds to me. Motivation for what? To never get cancer again? To run a marathon? To be the next winner on "The Voice"? What the hell does this statement even mean? I guess that's why this little nugget of "should" made it into the book. I have racked my brain over and over again trying to make real meaning out of this. Could it be motivation to be a better person? That would make sense. We can all work on being better versions of ourselves. But alas, I always draw a blank when it comes to this statement. Not helpful. Not at all. When I figure it out, I'll update my blog and let you know. Again, it ranks right up there with fear-induced statements, out of inadequacies in knowing what to say, out of complete ignorance about the whole process. For now, it's just one of many laughable paradoxes for me.

The only people who should be advising cancer patients about what they should and shouldn't do are trained medical professionals or those who have already traveled the road. Truth be told, even then, it's not always sound advice! When a survivor tells me to sleep when I need to, I sleep. When a well-trained medical professional shows me evidence that a particular treatment plan is the best path we have, I believe it. When someone brings me homemade chicken soup or a beet root supplement, I know for a fact it has cured something . . . but, cancer isn't it. The research just isn't complete yet. I stress *yet* because I welcome the day when that data is finalized and made widely available. There's a clear and distinct reason why we're told not to mix medications or supplements or foods with certain types of treatments. These are called contraindications. The same can be said about survival advice. Let the experts provide it. When you're traveling that road for the first time, you become reliant on them.

Along with "shoulda, woulda, coulda," comes guilt. This whole process brought to light a good heaping helping of guilt for me. Guilt about being quick to anger. Guilt about being a non-present, or over-present, or enabling, or neglectful parent. Guilt about being too fat, too thin, too right, too wrong, too nosy, too disconnected. Guilt about spending too much time devoted to work or not enough time devoted to work. Guilt about spending too much time with friends or not being a good enough friend. Guilt about having the "good cancer." Guilt about feeling healthy. Guilt about not being able to reach every survivor. Guilt about not being able to respond to every gift with a meaningful thank you. I wonder how much time I wasted quantifying my own pain and suffering where others around me had it far worse; my situation was clearly less severe because I happened to have decent insurance and a support system made of concrete and steel. *Well, you're strong and have Dave; you'll be okay.* Maybe it's a diagnosis that appears more promising than someone else's. So there's guilt that we don't deserve to have grief, to feel anger, to be anxious . . . that we should just "get over it" because we're so much more "okay" than someone else. I've had many friends state that if they jumped high enough, they could get over anything. I admired that approach wholeheartedly and carried it with me into this adventure. What I quickly learned was that cancer isn't just *anything*. Self-perceived, self-imposed guilt? Likely. Yet we're giving worth and power to what others may think when no one really has a clue about the depths of our pain or challenges. It's an apples and oranges process, folks. No one "does" cancer the same way. No one conquers adversity the same way. What I can say is, enough already! Guilt erodes your soul. We need to understand that guilt is often either self-imposed or learned behavior, but we have control over that. It's time to stop being card-carrying members of the "Shoulda, Woulda, Coulda Club."

The Interwebs

Ah, the Internet. The information age. Digital literacy. I work with educators and students of all ages about this very topic all over the country. And there I was, having to practice what I preached.

Going full throttle into research mode can be powerful. Knowledge is power, right? Well, we all are cognizant of the dangers of fake news. Just like fake news, not everything posted to the great World Wide Web is valid nor is it automatically factual. Shocker, I know. Inherently, we want answers. We want advice. We want to see what's happening with cancer research and treatment advancements. We want the data and statistics. We want to connect with others. I'm not sure how I can phrase this eloquently—DANGER! DANGER! DANGER! While connection to a support web of survivors and caretakers is paramount to trudging through the process, it can lead down a dark, naggy, whiny, scary path. Online spaces are ripe for discussion threads that only add to our angst. Survivor blogs and advice posts may be supportive and insightful, yet they may lack verified, factual content. Googling is one of the easiest things we can do, and trust me, I picked Google's brain more than I probably should have. *How long does fatigue last after treatment? What is the recurrence rate for Stage III breast cancer? What can I do for neuropathy? What are the best exercises for a breast surgery arm? What are the best supplements for breast cancer survivors?* This is just the tip of the iceberg. When I went through my search history, there were a dozen more leads. I found a lot of information. However, I spent an inordinate amount of time sifting through sources and contradictory information until I wasn't certain what to believe anymore. Yes, there are reputable, verified sources that exist. Finding them takes some serious and stealthy super sleuthing. Ask questions. Lots of them. In person. I was limited to only one thousand questions on each of my visits with my oncologist. There's a reason for that. More on that later.

I'm Fine

I understand grace. At some point in my childhood, I'm certain I was taught about the virtues of grace. Truth be told, I struggle with grace most of the time. It's better to put on a smiley face and pretend everything is okay. Power of positive thinking, right? Put on your "big girl pants," right? Big girls don't cry, right? My guess is that we females have all been told something to this effect at some point in our lives. I understand and honor those who can put on the pretty facade and let the world know they're fine. I'm not one of those individuals. Everyone deals with things differently. For me, grace was always somewhat of a mystery and often concealed itself behind a mask of fear. Ironically, I'm a newly minted "Most Improved Player" when it comes to grace under fire, but it took cancer to drag it out of me.

I'm fine: I was pretending to be okay when in all honesty, I was teetering on the edge of depression, which didn't do me much good. The Mental Health Foundation claims that the average person will say, "I'm fine" fourteen times a week, though just nineteen percent actually mean it. Not sure what defines an "average person," but this factoid doesn't surprise me at all, especially when it comes to casual chitchat about cancer. It's easier to be armed with an automated response rather than rehash every ache and pain and struggle. No one wants to converse with a "Debbie Downer." (SNL. Google it—Rachel Dratch is hilarious as she crushes souls). "I'm fine" isolates. It turns out I was experiencing true, clinically diagnosed depression. *Maybe everyone would be better off without me. No one needs to see me. No one wants to hear about my progress. There's really nothing worth living for anymore. I'm just a burden.* That's when I knew it was real. I had never encountered this complete despondency and despair before in my life. Ever. It opened my eyes and taught me empathy for those who deal with depression on a daily basis. Every hour of the day. Anxiety is one thing. Depression is a completely different monster. "I'm fine" becomes a defense mechanism . . . to get away from the "C" word, to not talk about it, to not deal with it. But it just doesn't work.

My job affords me the privilege of working with all types of educators across our state to help them incorporate technology in their classrooms. I enjoy experimenting with applications in an attempt to leverage them for productivity and teaching and learning. One app I use frequently is the Voxer app, which is a walkie-talkie app you can use on your phone. I initially used it to join an international education book study group. I then connected with others in the space. It was a great way to communicate with my two sisters, especially when it came to matters like planning family gatherings, sharing ideas, and supporting each other. Then, when two of my closest friends moved, we used it as a way to stay connected. Additionally, I joined a few more chat circles with other friends, and it turned out to be one of the most impactful types of support I ever experienced. These spaces allowed all of us to "not be fine." I remember sobbing until I couldn't speak, so texting was a great way to connect when I was completely broken. I had one friend who reached out every couple of weeks when she knew I would be in the "valleys" of my chemo journey. She would leave me "pick-me-up" messages, mostly sharing stories of what her middle schoolers did that day. She knew my spirits would immediately lift with stories about her students. I normally don't jump on any specific device or app bandwagons, but having people within a fingertip's reach was powerful. I leaned on these friends so much when I wasn't fine. Each in their own unique ways, they made it possible for me to return to "I'm fine" without my nose growing. Because of them, I plodded my way back to an authentic "I'm fine."

I'm pretty much an open book. Likely, an oversharer by some standards. I choose to share my story openly because if someone can gain some miniscule morsel of insight or inspiration or some little nugget worth knowing, it's worth it. If nothing else, I want anyone trudging through any type of crapfest to completely and unequivocally soak in these three things: a) you are not alone, b) someone else "gets it", and c) it is perfectly okay to be "not okay." It's such a struggle. Sometimes just having a sounding board is all we need, someone to lend an ear, maybe a word of advice, or perhaps pull you completely back from the ledge to get your feet firmly planted once again so you can resume living your life. We want to sprint back into a regular work routine and establish a doable work-life balance, engage in social interactions, yet deal with a pesky social anxiety dichotomy—wanting to hide and lick our wounds but desperately wanting to interact with those who mean the most. I can only imagine that following an exceptionally brutal battle, Amazons would return to their beloved homeland, evaluate casualties, analyze strategy, mourn losses together (from what I read, there was wild, unabashed dancing, chanting, and imbibing of potent drink and herbs around fires), and then regroup, sharpen spears and swords, and redress their trusty steeds for the next impending battle. That's what cancer does. It knocks you down, you get a bit of a respite of some normalish, and then the aftermath offers up a new set of mini battles to face.

See what I mean by whiplash?

__The card face said this, " We've been through a lot together, and most of it was your fault."__

Kaye,

I just couldn't resist—but the truth is—probably not your fault! (*smiles.) You are my "fuel," my inspiration, my "hope" to always better myself and soldier on when the going gets tough (crying, happy, proud, too!) Please know I think about you <u>every day</u>—pray every morning for that serenity, courage, and wisdom we so often refer to in our chats.

I'm so proud to be your friend. You are rock solid, one of the strongest women I know and love, and you've got this! I love ya, gal! I'm there for you, in twenty-four hours, if needed!

Much love,

A.R.

Chapter 10: The Seasoning of a Resilient Warrior

{
Skill and confidence are an unconquered army.
~George Herbert~
}

Knowledge

It's vital to have good, solid, valid knowledge from reliable sources. Survivors I know are uber cautious about making your cancer seem like theirs. That's because, until you've slipped on cancer shoes and slogged through it yourself, it's impossible to understand that every single cancer diagnosis is unique. Yes, when a woman walks into the grocery store bald as a cue ball, people assume it's breast cancer, well, because breast cancer chemo drugs cause alopecia. Knowing that every cancer diagnosis is unique to each person is an eye-opener. At least, it was for me. I believe revisiting the whole "know it all" of my past self was a result of a self-imposed inadequacy of never knowing enough. Never being enough. Never doing enough. Enough already. We'll never know enough, and information changes in a blink of an eye. That's why learning never ends. What worked twenty years ago—heck, even ten years ago—may not be as effective today. The same applies to any adversity. Whether it's depression, divorce, or dieting, there's a wealth of information we can draw from valid sources that is more about self-advocacy and continuous learning than anything else. Never stop learning! Know where you get your information; consider the source, as they say. Because we are unique in the information we seek, encourage others to steer their own learning as well. In this case, knowledge can be power!

Resilience Isn't Resistance

Do one thing every day that scares you.
~Eleanor Roosevelt~

Mrs. Roosevelt's words have been posted on everything from my social media spaces to my journal. I wonder what her intentions were with this little pearl of wisdom. Any time someone experiences a life adversity, whether it be a bitter divorce trial or watching a child in the hospital or the challenges about what to do with your career or how to pay the bills—every day, that scary thing breaks you down . . . and ultimately and hopefully, builds you back up, adding a layer or two of armor and making you more resilient than you ever thought possible to face any battle just like any warrior princess worth her salt. Every day of this process is scary. I made the mistake of believing that resisting connection, resisting advice, resisting assistance would help me. I thought it made me stronger. Warrior princesses don't need a helping hand, for crying out loud. "Caving in" would only make me weaker. The higher I built the wall, the more I would be protected and be able to "just do this on my own." Ginormous errors in logic. When we are smack-dab in the middle of fighting, whatever it may be, we spend all that energy on unintentionally hurting ourselves instead of embracing all that is good to strengthen our resolve, our resilience. I thought I could bury my pain, all the pain, by numbing it. Whether that meant shutting down emotionally or popping open a bottle of wine or striking a warrior pose for every single little thing that mentally challenged me, I did everything I could to bury the pain. That was empty-headed.

Resilience is trudging through the muck. Resilience is accepting your reality. Resilience is wrapping your noodle around what you need to do to move forward . . . then doing it. Resilience is resistance to painting on a Stepford wife facade of perfection—of perfectly pressed clothes, perfectly quaffed hair, perfectly applied makeup, and pretending everything is hunky-dory perfect. Rather, take a tenacious approach to adversity—this is where we are, this is reality, there are problems, so now let's brainstorm possible strategies to cope and get through this mess. Resilience is sometimes going rogue when you need to. Resilience is recognizing when you need help. Resilience is knowing what you need and going after it. Resilience is taking a moment to lick our wounds. Resilience is making conscious decisions whether or not to go bald, go flat, go forward. Resilience is truly a choice. Every single element of resilience circles back to my Amazon heroines. Everything they did, they did out of resilience. They knew their potential fate yet they faced their adversity head-on, all with the endgame of protecting each other, protecting their territory, and protecting their existence. I guess that's a gigantic reason why this mythology resonates with me. Myth or reality, they teach us powerful lessons.

Blog Post: Suck it Up, Cupcake

What is resilience anyway?

Is it a stiff upper lip?

Is it puppy dogs and unicorns?

Is it "walking on sunshine" on the outside when everything on the inside is a discombobulated pile of mysterious crap?

Is it some tough guy/girl arrogance with an impervious facade?

I'm not sure anymore.

Let's circle back to resilience. Life happens. Curveballs happen. Bitch slaps—sledgehammer style—happen.

The funny thought I have is that we try so hard to "teach" our children resilience, but to what end? Parents, teachers, grands, extended family members, community leaders, clergy, coaches. You name it. We're here for our kids. The world's not fair. We need to teach them how to be tougher, right? It's only recently dawned on me how futile this noble endeavor can be.

Who would want their kids to experience any type of abuse, be it substance, verbal, physical, sexual, or anything else? Who would want their kids to deal with absent or neglectful parents? Who would place them in harm's way to satisfy their own ambitions and/or egos? Who would ever think it's okay to let our kids experience cyberbullying, or playground bullying, or any other form of bullying? No one I can think of, anyway. The funny thing is that in order to be resilient, we must experience some pretty harsh junk. We can't be taught it . . . until we're dead center in the middle of a life smackdown. The same goes for our kids. What can we do? Simply and sadly, all we can do is share our experiences, explain how we have learned from them, and model resilience.

Resilience comes from, and only from, experience. As people who want the best for the next generation, we spend our lifetimes devoted to ensuring our kids don't experience some of the struggles we did growing up. What does that do? How on Earth does that prepare them to deal with authentic, real life struggles? We can't possibly take into account, or pre-plan, for what the next generations will encounter. How can we ever plan for the tragic death of a loved one? How can we possibly prepare for a life-threatening illness? Miscarriage? Divorce? The texting driver swerving over the centerline into oncoming traffic? The bigotry and blatant racism we've somehow gotten sucked into? How can we possibly be ready for any of this? Thing is, these things happen every day . . . and how we encounter and react to them varies with each one of us—some reactions are destructive, and some are productive.

Oprah Winfrey once said, "Where there is no struggle, there is no strength." While none of us put out a welcome mat inviting struggle into our lives, the struggles show up and crash our perfectly planned life party nonetheless. And let's be honest, when most of us wail, "The struggle is real," it's really first-world problems we're dealing with. Yep. Guilty, as charged.

I've been reflecting a lot about all of this over the year we're calling, "The Reset Year." Suddenly, all the "struggles" I thought I had disappeared. I stopped obsessing over them. I stopped lamenting about them. They faded to black and now I don't even remember what my big, hairy, greasy "struggles" were in the first place.

Resilience jumps at the chance to say, "Alrighty then. This is where we are. So what? Now what?"

Resilience makes you seek solutions, answers, and relief.

Resilience helps you smile when you need to and allows you to cry when you have to. Resilience is pinpoint clarity about all things important. (And the crap that isn't.)

Resilience drops all the other stuff off the highest rooftop you can find and watches it go SPLAT on the pavement below.

Resilience is dirty. It's messy. It doesn't come in neat, colorful packaging. It's ugly. It's truth. It's liberating.

Resilience, or the best definition I can come up with, is accepting things over which we have zero, zilch, nada control and taking a painful yet necessary look in the mirror, then screaming at the top of our lungs, "Suck it up, Cupcake!"

Who Rescued Whom?

Dave and I are dog people. We've always had dogs. Most times, multiple dogs. That said, we've never had inside dogs. Nope. No dog hair in the house. No dog claws scuffing up our hardwoods or leather furniture. No random bouts of uncontrolled bowel movements left for us to step in. Nope. All that stayed outside where it belonged.

Enter this goldish-orange beagle-pit shelter puppy. Our daughter, also a lover of animals, fell in love with her and picked her up at a local shelter, mostly I think to help remedy some feelings about not being with her kids all the time because of her sudden divorce and subsequent joint custody of them. No one could blame her. It's quiet around the house when the kids are gone. Long story short, living arrangements at the time were not conducive to having a puppy . . . sooooooo, could Geneva "hang out" with us until she found a bigger and better yard for her to run around in? Hang out for a while? Sure thing. We are dog people, after all.

Well, this fifty-pound lap dog, with all her golden hairs of love dropped everywhere, ultimately became the newest member of the family. I could see why Ashley picked her. She's smart and has a feisty, loving personality. Dogs' intuition when something is wrong is something I'll never understand but something for which I'm forever grateful. Geneva, and all of her rambunctious energy, was surprisingly delicate with me while I recovered from surgery. She watched me sleep when I needed to sleep. To aid in rest and recovery, I often slept in a reclining chair in our living room. It made healing more comfortable to be semi-seated as opposed to horizontal in our bed. Routinely, Geneva invited herself to our laps, because well, doesn't everyone need a fifty-pound lap dog? She's definitely a cuddler. Without delay, she found her place on the sofa, where we had placed a blanket so her profuse shedding wouldn't destroy it. It was conveniently located just to the left of my recovery chair. Occasionally, she would leap onto my lap. Ironically, she only did this after I healed. She obediently watched me rest when I was sliced up, combatting fatigue from chemo, or blistering from radiation. She knew! She always knew! We went for walks together when it was time to get moving again, and she never yanked her leash like she normally did when we walked. She is a beagle, after all. You can't deny the impressive talent of a beagle's nose. I cannot imagine where I would be mentally or emotionally without her. Never saying a word, she understood absolutely everything that was going on. I understand canine therapy is not for everyone. Not everyone savors a good slobber session with a pooch. There's just something about an animal's unconditional love that can cure most of what ails us. At least, this was the case for me. Every day, it was as if she was saying, "I've got you, Mom . . . now, let's have a treat!" She can't be our family member without an affinity for food. Anyone who wants to argue that dogs don't have souls, I'm up for a lively conversation!

Balance and Purpose

When adversity hits, balance is critical. Let's face it, the whole life-work-leisure balance gets blown out of whack. The whole complicated, yet necessary, rest-nutrition-movement triangle of healthy living morphs into a bloated, mangled trapezoid. And, when we get out of balance, fear creeps through the cracks in our balance beams. The rush to return to any sense of normalish seems in vain. That's when we feel overwhelmed. As a matter of fact, I've banned that word—*normal*—forever from my vocabulary. Who am I kidding? Nothing will ever be normal again. Ever. So, I settle on normalish. I can live with normalish. I'm fairly certain the Amazons felt fear. I'm certain they pondered what normalish looked like after defeat, death, and devastation. We just never see it played out in the annals of lore or on the big screens of Hollywood.

Then, there's purpose. Granted, not everything we do is going to be super purposeful. It's life. However, increasing studies link a sense of purpose to living longer. Purpose and burnout are directly related. When we lose connection with our original intention or purpose, we lose balance, and we burnout. If we infuse everything we do, or at least most of what we do, with meaning, we bring a deeper value into our routine, day-to-day activities. This doesn't mean we need to embark on a full life makeover, but cancer and adversity force us to rethink and realign our dots for more purposeful connection. When the clouds dissipate, we can begin to engage in practices that allow purpose to reignite. I learned to play the piano again. Music soothes my soul, and it's been years since I've played. I called up a local piano tuner, dusted off some old sheets of music and cracked my knuckles as I sat down in front of the ivory keys. I stopped worrying about the "cost" of everything and shifted my thinking to the "cost" of not doing something. Like anything worth doing, it's not always easy. Yes, today might have been hard, but we've got this.

Connection to others aids with balance. You can verbally vomit all your woes to those who understand and want desperately to help you. You can also connect yourself to causes worth your energy and those that fill your soul. That worked for me. I have a few endeavors currently in the works to bring more support and kinship to those struggling with cancers (and other adversities) to more rural, regional centers. We have some pretty amazing medical facilities and professionals in our neck of the woods, and for that, we are so incredibly fortunate. However, someone needing some serious, compassionate conversation and support shouldn't have to drive an hour or more one way to receive it. Someone yearning to learn more about impactful mindfulness practice should be able to access it where they are, when they need it. We need access to support in outreach areas. This is my purpose. Stay tuned.

Advocacy

Remember when I was limited to only one thousand questions per medical visit? That goes for life *after* cancer, too. So many questions. A pervasive misconception exists that once you've completed the treatment path, there are no more steps. You're done. I believed it. Until I got there. Advocacy for self, advocacy for others—it never ends. I found myself somewhat discontented, somewhat curious to know more, to more fully understand my situation, so I asked. I asked a lot. It seems like the advice, research, and support abound as we begin a journey with cancer. In times of darkness, we need light. Light comes in answers, in direction, in hope. This is what I call my "So What? Now What?" phase. Ask questions, press issues, ask for data, research, proof . . . even if it's anecdotal. At the same time, be prepared to share data, *be* the proof, dig deep into becoming your own best advocate or advocate for other thrivers. I typically did this, as noted ad nauseum, out of anger. Maybe it was fear. I'm no stranger to equating advocacy to fighting. That's the warrior princess way, after all. Turns out, it really has nothing to do with anger. It has everything to do with passion, compassion, and determination to hold your head high for what you know in your gut to be right, to be true, to be necessary. Advocacy must continue far beyond the end of the tunnel.

More than once in my life I've been called uncoachable. Through some incredibly dedicated advocacy and persistence, a wellness colleague found a way to break through the armor and help me see things from a different perspective. It took tears, it took time, and it took tenacity in true teamwork fashion to unearth the core of this uncoachable guise I had carried with me since tweenhood. Her advocacy for my life, her determination to help me uncover all the good stuff have inspired me to do the same for others. The uncoachable armor was just that—armor. So I advocate . . . almost annoyingly. *Have you checked your tatas this month? Over fifty? How about that colonoscopy appointment? Have you heard about gut health? Wanna go for a quick jaunt around the office for a brain break? Do you know your numbers? (cholesterol, blood pressure, glucose levels, etc.)* I do this regularly. I'm certain I am a nuisance. I'm fine with that. But maybe one day they'll thank me!

As I noted before, throughout these efforts, one very specific topic keeps bubbling to the top of my purpose priority list. Living in a rural area and having amazing and progressive health care only an hour from our home, I feel fortunate. Fortunate beyond words. Cancer support group meetings were offered on Wednesday nights at 6:30. *This is great,* I thought. I welcomed the opportunity to connect with and learn from others. Who wouldn't need or want to hear words of encouragement, words of wisdom, words of like-minded compassion. My issue was the distance. *An hour-plus away?! Were there any support groups closer to where I lived?*

Were there any regional centers I could attend? I searched. I inquired. Nope. Nothing. I could always travel an hour one way, on a weeknight, when I was clearly at my lowest point both physically and emotionally, and then drive home and attempt to snag a few hours of sleep before the next day. This seemed so peculiar to me, that in this day and age of access to regional health care for the *physical* portion of treating cancer, there was little to nothing locally available to support the *emotional* struggles of cancer . . . for patient or caregiver. It bothers me to this day. Enter my most recent advocacy efforts. A number of cancer survivors I've met through social media and other advocacy connections are working with me to create regional support opportunities. It's a work in progress and a labor of love. This is a huge, gaping mental health hole in the treatment of cancer, and this dogged warrior princess is ready for battle to bring these centers to life.

Ironically, advocacy for others parallels advocacy for self. Weaving my cancer journey into the threads of my education skill set, I've ventured into survive-to-thrive workshops with not only survivors but also with others affected by a cancer diagnosis. It's not enough to be on the "survivor list." It's important to continue to grow, the "so what, now what" stage of kicking cancer in the backside. I've taken coaching classes and discovered professional networking opportunities to gain new knowledge and skills to fulfill this purpose. That's the funny thing with advocacy. Once you start, it often thrusts you headfirst into purpose. In the middle of the darkness, we ask, "Why am I even here? What if I wouldn't have done the self-exam? What if I had been diagnosed with a later stage and it had spread? What's next? How can others grow through my struggle? So what? Now what?" These are just a sampling of questions that we as cancer survivors may have, and with consistent advocacy and growth of our networks, we can find solidarity and humanity through others. Warriors build their armies. Warriors continue to support each other through any battle, big or small.

Kaye,

You are a very special person to all. We always look forward to hearing your laugh and seeing your smile at the lake! Sending you a little treat* to keep you warm! Keep the faith. We will keep you and Dave in our prayers!

Hugs,

C and B

*The little "treat" was a gorgeous, hand-crocheted prayer shawl, something I saw too many times in my visits to the infusion center during chemo. It adorns our guest room so the comfort and positivity it once shined on me can be shared with our guests.

Chapter 11: The Power of Sisterhood: Back to Good Again

> *The wheel is come full circle.*
> *~William Shakespeare~*

More whiplash. The good, the bad, and the ugly . . . and back to good again. There's no way to make cancer "un-ugly" or "un-bad." As my wonderful, talented oncologist repeatedly told me, to make cancer go away, hopefully forever, we:

- CUT IT (surgery)
- POISON IT (chemo)
- BURN IT (radiation)
- STARVE IT (subsequent hormone therapy lasting anywhere from five to ten years)

Now it's all well and good that cancer is defeated through these battle strategies. The thing is, defeat happens to our hearts and other vital organs, too. Our bodies, minds, and souls are cut, poisoned, burned, and starved during the course of treatment. It's bad. And, it's ugly. While we have powerful treatments to get rid of cancer once and for all, we run the risk of killing healthy cells doing their things inside. It's a risk. And risk is scary. Another battle.

The good. What "good" could possibly come from cancer. You know? As I said before, when I was first diagnosed, my nurse navigators assured me that, believe it or not, cancer survivors say that this phoenix of positivity arises from the ashes of cancer battles. That it is actually a gift. *You have GOT to be kidding me. How can anything POSITIVE come from this?!* I've just been informed I have something deadly wreaking havoc inside my body. I'm being told I'm going to be sliced up, filled full of poison, and fried. And all of this is going to rob well over a year (once again, I am fully aware that others have been through far worse for far longer) from my life, and I am never going to be the same again. Ever. How the hell is something positive ever going to rise from this? How?

Fellow warrior/survivor/thriver sisters who shared their nigglings about life after breast cancer gave me hope. They resonated deep within me when I needed them most. Their words gave me hope. Their words opened my mind. I gained fresh perspective and assurance from this profound sisterhood. Maybe there was something good about all of this after all? Just maybe.

Their words are powerful and can serve as guidance for any of us traveling a road wrought with challenge and adversity:

"I considered myself a survivor, not a victim. I think about recurrence, but it no longer consumes me. I do not fear death, nor do I fear life after having breast cancer. My life will never be the same as before, but any negative that breast cancer has brought has been matched by positives." ~ H.B.

"Once I overcame breast cancer, I wasn't afraid of anything anymore." ~ M.E.

"The most important thing about cancer is learning you can say no to others. I couldn't before. I couldn't say no to my kids. I couldn't say no to my spouse, but I can say no now. It's a very important thing to be able to do." ~ E.B.

"The only person who can save you is you: That was going to be the thing that informed the rest of my life." ~ S.C.

"There comes a time after you grieve your losses when you have to choose if you want to live your life as a memorial service around the event or learn from the horrible things sent your way and build a new and even better life." ~B.H.

If I *had* to thank cancer for something, it was this expanding treasury of parallel stories with other survivors, in sisterhood. Oddly enough, those parallels became perpendicular, creating an unintentional, but welcomed, intersection of inspiration, growth, and gratitude. That's where the magic happened. Captain Obvious here: I'm not there. Yet. I have no doubt I'll arrive there someday. I'm just taking my own sweet time arriving.

One bad and ugly that needs to be addressed is the anxiety that accompanies adversity and trauma. For me, it was the onslaught of panic attacks that ensued long after diagnosis, treatment, and maintenance. With no known reason. I had no clue what brought these on. I sought high and low to identify triggers, with little to no luck. Come to learn I had bouts of what is called generalized anxiety disorder (GAD), a condition that makes you feel anxious and worried about everyday things or seemingly nothing at all. I knew my worries were often unrealistic, but that didn't make them easier to deal with. Anxiety's intense symptoms can last for long periods of time. I needed to address this and seek help . . . another skill I can file under "work in progress."

It's important to understand that like losing a loved one or suffering a tragedy of a different flavor, cancer survivors go through all the stages of grief. My question is why these little coping nuggets were never shared with me? Why did I have to seek these out on my own? More importantly, why is this not being addressed with other cancer patients/survivors/caretakers? Especially in rural, more regional areas. Being reminded of this makes me more eager than ever to increase awareness. We need more regional support services, plain and simple. We have work to do. The battle rages on.

The Aftermath

In the wake of the most serious storms, there is an aftermath. Some storms leave rubbish; some leave complete ruin. That said, the sun eventually shines, scars heal, and fatigue lessens. It's necessary to clear the rubble in order for new growth to flourish. Much like recovering from a natural disaster, the aftermath of cancer is messy, it takes times, and no one can do it alone. Not even warrior princesses.

Aftermath includes a whole lot of breathholding. You hold your breath through the whole process of follow-up appointments and subsequent tests. Additional scans are ordered to ensure that yes, the beast is indeed gone. You hold your breath until the results come in. Then, every follow up appointment, the breathholding continues. You hold your breath when the out-of-pocket bills come. You hold your breath when your white blood cell counts drop dramatically, turning someone who used to play in flower garden dirt regularly into a bonafide germaphobe—and not in a pleasant way. It doesn't consume everyday thinking, but like a bad rash or weeds that invade that beautiful flower garden, it just keeps popping up. Though reduced in intensity, the whiplash continues.

Have you ever been so neck-deep in the quagmire that it's nearly impossible to see any flicker of light at the end of an endless tunnel? This is all part of the topsy-turvy roller coaster of adversity aftermath. Then, there it is. The gift. The purpose. The clarity that those brave souls before me alluded to. The clarity that, up until now, had been lost in the muck for me. Through my commiserations, it dawned on me what I needed to do. Sometimes, when we're seeking our purpose, we try so hard . . . too hard. We just need to be still. It will come to you when you aren't looking. The process, or proper procedure even, is difficult to put into words, but it's true that in darkness, there is light. In nothingness, there is purpose. That's part of the aftermath of whiplash, too.

I completely underestimated the toll that being blindsided would take on me. I was prepared for surgery. I was prepared for treatment. I read everything I could get my hands on when I was first diagnosed. But nothing adequately prepared me for that otherwise uneventful morning when I found myself standing in front of the mirror. I blinked at my new body and bravely wrapped my head around my new shapes, missing pieces, and unruly zaps of random pain. It was not like those pre-cancer days of bemoaning about not having anything to wear. It was my new reality. As I racked my brain, I realized there was limited information in my research that talked about living life after a mastectomy.

The first thing I noticed following a long healing process was that traditional lingerie no longer fit me. It was a slap in the face. There would be no more Victoria's Secret® moments of lingerie admiration. It was more like lingerie survival mode. I had no idea that putting something as simple as a bra on could be so challenging. I wish I had known this ahead of time. I walked into my closet, like I did on any given morning. Sifting through the hangers of tops, bottoms, dresses, fabrics. No one forewarns you that certain fabrics are going to feel like sandpaper grating against your numb, scar-adorned skin. I tried to remain positive and jovial.

"Heck, you're getting perky boobs out of this thing!" friends would remind me. They knew where my humor boundaries were at this point, and it was comical . . . most of the time.

Ummm, no. I've never had a boob job, but I'm quite certain this is nothing like it. The density, shape, and consistency of implants are vastly different than that of normal tissue, and radiation completely altered my skin and muscle on my right side into tightened leather. And let's not even get started on the nipple conversation. There's also the lopsidedness no one mentioned. Okay, I take that back. I was told that there would be "shifting," and I am absolutely, 100 percent satisfied with the crazy skills of my plastic reconstructive surgeon. Again, I had to discover a new "normalish" when it came to wardrobe. I certainly could have used some guidance on polyester as your frenemy (easy on the wallet, but itchy like chicken pox on scar tissue) situation. So, now I'm gearing up for comfort. When I'm comfortable, I'm productive and pleasant to be around. Anyone want to come to my house for a rummage sale? Lots of bras to sell!

There's something cyclical about all of this. I think, as survivors and warriors, our thinking revolves around being DONE. Once the treatment is completed, we are DONE. Every battle round takes its time. They also require patience. The aftermath is full of "never befores." That's where the "new normal" adage comes from. Again, not a big fan. There's nothing normal about any of this. The aftermath includes living with neuropathy. It includes numerous follow-up medical appointments. Spontaneous bouts of fears and tears, panic attacks based in irrational thought, are part and parcel of the aftermath. Fear triggers sweating, heart palpitations, unpredictable waterworks, and it all takes you by surprise. *Ghhheeeeeezzz! Where the hell did that come from?* Little stressors of everyday life take on a whole new life of their own. With the follow-up testing, the scans, the blood work, the probing . . . all of these little battles seem endless, when in reality, perspective changes. Because of all the follow-up exams, all of the poking and prodding, I have a much clearer understanding of the way my body works. I understand my blood counts. I know what's going on . . . and thankfully, not going on . . . everywhere else in my body. I think that's where perspective is everything. Yes, these can weigh heavily on your heart, but seeing them in a positive, preventative light makes all the difference in the world!

Truth be told, I had never considered this aftermath before. I was solely focused on finishing and surviving through this crappy stuff. I never took into account that the aftermath is also an integral part of the process. The fatigue, physical reboot, clothes and fabrics not fitting right on new skin, lopsidedness, financial toll—all of these factors and many more made us think back to the days of choosing more thriftily—prepping and eating more at home, fewer road trips, simpler pleasures, and living with intention. Through these forced perspective shifts in thinking and some innovations in living, we take back control. We can be future focused, regardless of what the future might hold and wrap our heads around "normalish" when we don't even know what normal is anymore. We can be honest and vulnerable about acknowledging fatigue, anxiety, and fear. We just need to harness it, especially when that harness digs deep into our hands, leaving blisters and slices. Warriors can shift perspective. Not always easily, but they can. Warriors have this power. *We* have that power. We all do.

Kacee,

Read your email. Holy cow! So sorry your test results came out so negatively, but it will all work out. You're a rare breed, with spirit and spunk, so I know you will be okay. You're young and shouldn't have to spend valuable time fighting this, but we don't always get to choose our paths, I guess. You have a phenomenal support team, but you can always use a few more—so please know I am in your corner, and so is God. Prayers are the most important part of your fight, and you'll have endless sessions of them from us.

God Bless!

Love,

L.P.

Chapter 12: Embracing the Big, Bad New Normal

{ *There is no normality in life.*
~Helena Bonham Carter~ }

Nobody invites adversity into their lives. It isn't like we go out there and *look* for bad stuff to happen. Yet, it happens. For some unfortunate souls, it happens more than it should. So, what do we do? How do we not spend the rest of our lives balled up in the fetal position, locking our doors—and our hearts, in some cases—and disconnecting from the world, or even from reality?

The reality is that there will never be *normal* again. It's a cliché that says we, as survivors of any kind of life-altering adversity, need to find our "new normal." Well, in case you missed the memo, there is no normal. Never again. I will never have my breasts again. I will never have organs and innards untouched by vicious poisons or that burned until I bled. I will never go to sleep without tingling and tightening in my right hand. I will never go have my labs drawn thinking everything will be hunky-dory. I will never stop worrying whether this devil lurks somewhere else in my body.

So, we land on "normalish" as the new standard of life.

In true warrior princess fashion, circling back to normalish needed to start with a proclamation. Turning fifty was kind of a big deal for me. I had such big plans when I crossed that half-century mark. As you can imagine, cancer wasn't remotely part of that vision. Cancer detoured me for a year and some change. Cancer delayed my big, hairy, #50-at-50 bucket list. I even had a hashtag, for Pete's sake! Challenges and adversity may force you to hit the pause button. That doesn't mean we can't pick up the pieces and move forward, dusting off the grime from our eyes and wiping the blood from our wounds. That's what warrior princesses do; they pick up their shields and swords when they get knocked down, bang out the kinks in the armor, and prepare for battle again.

Blog Post: Reset Button

When I turned fifty in 2016, like most people my age, I created a grandiose bucket list. I planned to hashtag it with #50-at-50 . . . fifty things I normally wouldn't do, but always wanted a reason to. I wanted to do things that scared the crap out of me (skydiving), try foods that normally made me squeamish (squid), or visit somewhere that would enlighten my soul (Tibet). Get this all done before October 19, 2017.

Well? Today's October 19, 2017, and I turn fifty-one. At 7:03 p.m., to be exact, so there's still time, right? Nah, I'm heading to my eighteenth radiation treatment after work. So much for that hashtag . . .

PROCLAMATION: I hereby anoint the remainder of 2017

(and much of 2018) as my "Reset Year." The year of the pause button. The year of doing something that not only scared me a little more than a little but also crushed me into a million teeny tiny shards only to refashion, repurpose, and revitalize a whole new, better (albeit bent and cracked) version of me.

I never made it to Tibet, yet my soul has been enlightened and recharged repeatedly this year by connections made with other survivors and supporters, reconnections with dear (I won't say *old*) friends, and new connections made . . . and I never had to leave home thanks to social media and some pretty powerful networks. I've cried more this year than the previous fifty combined, and, most importantly, I've learned, at this half-century mark, about what really matters. Not some silly hashtag, not some inspirational YouTube video, not the amount of likes, followers, or click-throughs.

As with any opportunity for learning, I've collected a few "adversity" nuggets to share:

- One never gets to be "done" with cancer (again, insert your own adversity here) journey. It just continues, much like the backroads of the gorgeous western Wisconsin countryside, swerving along the way. It can be a beautiful ride; it can give you whiplash and make you lose your lunch. There's definitely a destination, but the journey never ends. You never "get over" having cancer; you simply get through it . . . hopefully. It's truly a matter of seeking "what's next?"
- I have it so much better than some. The hair on the back

of my neck prickles when I think about the health care conversations people are having every day about cancer. I have a support network larger than most, and for that I'm reminded daily about how grateful I should be. It makes me almost sicker to see people alone in the waiting rooms. It makes me cringe when I see how the almighty dollar and greed impact people's lives. What can we do to lift each other up? What can we do to ensure quality of life for as many as we can?

- No matter how severe the adversity, we always get two choices: get bitter, or get better. And as always, I choose the latter.
- There's no need to have all the answers or be able to fix everything, especially if they're not even broken. Believing this can kill you.

That said, I'm bidding this year good riddance—ahead of time because my mom would always say, "If you can't be on time, be early." (Thanks, Mom!)

I'd say it's been real, but then my nose would grow, and I'd be struck by lightning.

It's been a gigantic cluster.

It's been an eye-opener.

It's been so excruciatingly painful.

And . . .

It's almost time to hit the reset button.

So, what happens next? Where do we go from here when we've been through hell and back?

A new hashtag, of course!

Cheers to Happy Reset Year!

#51Reset

Part of my reset is remembering that I am an Amazon warrior. Throughout my life, I've refused to be defined by my circumstances. I was a teen mother. Yes, I understood the potential ramifications. I was made acutely and frequently aware of the statistics. Heck, my high school guidance counselor flat out told me I would likely not graduate from college because I was raising a child. (Ahem, women do this all the time, mister.) I would not succumb to these archaic statistics. I experienced a whole myriad of abuses throughout my childhood and developmental years. I never once considered myself a victim. Instead, I clutched rather tightly to the belief that *what doesn't kills you only makes you stronger*. And, it has. I encourage others to reflect and celebrate how much strength they have cultivated through their bouts with adversity. The same applies to my journey with cancer. I am hesitant to call myself a survivor. The nurses told me that the minute a woman is diagnosed, she becomes a survivor. Wait. What?! I had a hell of a long path to travel before I could clang the survivor gong. I prefer thriving. It is not enough to merely survive trauma, adversity, turmoil, or a life-threatening diagnosis. We must thrive. And that is my intention: survivor to thriver. I always find a way. I land on my feet. Sometimes I stumble and trudge through mud and get insanely filthy, cut up, and battered, but I eventually land on my feet. I stand up. The question now is, "How can I help others discover that grit in themselves to stand back up again after they've been pummeled to the ground? How can I help them be powerful warriors?"

Now, there are days I completely forget about ever having cancer. Even though I falter at times to maintain a perfectly perpetual perkiness about adversity and life in general, I firmly believe in the power of positive thinking (but not unicorn glitter farts, remember). Becoming so engrossed with purposeful work that matters makes me forget about cancer for that moment. Supporting others' dreams and ensuring that the gift of clarity from a cancer journey is put to good use makes me forget about cancer. Doing what makes my mind, my body, and my soul content makes me forget about cancer. Such are the days I work with youth. Such are the days I collaborate with like-minded colleagues and those who challenge the way I think. Such are the days digging in the dirt, planting seeds, and watching them grow. Such are the days encouraging our children and grandchildren to embrace a love of all things nature, witnessing miracles that happen every single day, and experiencing transformation of individuals, both young and old, as they reach for life goals. Such are the days I can go longer, stretch farther, dig deeper, and sleep more soundly. Such are the days to celebrate life, celebrate connection, and celebrate successes, no matter how big or how small. The days when setbacks, chronic pain, and meaningless challenges are overshadowed and silenced. Those are the days I forget about breast cancer. My point is, days like this exist. Embrace them. They help open the window to normalish again.

Even if "normal" eludes us forever, we persevere. We come full circle. We hit the reset button. We're alive. We're vertical (most days!). We're moving forward—I hope! It's that circling back to what truly matters that becomes the new focus. And what really does matter, anyway? I think we all ask ourselves this question time and time again, regardless of the severity of adversity. It's that renewed focus on what truly matters that helps us determine a "new normal." The beautiful thing is that now, once we emerge from the darkness, *we* hold the power. We can regain the control. We also can have the courage to admit we are indeed, vulnerable. We can admit openly that we continue to strive to be the best version of ourselves each and every day. We can admit when we slide. We can call the shots when we transition from surviving to thriving . . . as long as we're moving forward. We can define "normal." We have that power. Finding normal again is like trudging through a forest, peeling through the layers of trees, weeds, bushes, and brambles. It's confusing. We get lost at times. We think we're on the right path, things feel "normal," and then all of a sudden, we're stuck in the brambles again and we get all cut up, and we're suddenly askew. The goal is to cultivate more good days, more smiles, and more bravery, daring to live a life that is rich and full.

I like connecting dots, making ideas connect to each other, creating a network of learning, of sorts. One of my most profound dot connections comes from my own continuous learning efforts and something I stumbled on called the Triad of Wellness: Emotional, Nutritional, Physical—keys to living well. Reverse the focus a bit—get yourself well so you can be there for others. Rest! Water! Healthful nutrition choices—eating for energy. Keeping substances that drain energy, motivation, and clarity at a distance. With neuropathy, especially, the new normal where the Triad of Wellness takes on a whole new meaning when it comes to the importance of gut health and getting in those healthy supplements.

For those who have never been diagnosed with cancer, this can be a lifelong practice, too. It doesn't guarantee that you'll never get cancer, mind you. Anything can happen to anyone at any time. Didn't someone say the only guarantees in life are death and taxes? But why not take care of yourself when you can?

I find it ironic that the very first things I blogged about when I started this journey pretty much sum up, well, everything.

Blog Post: I Don't Do Vulnerable

I've never been one to open the door to vulnerability. Being vulnerable has always been somewhat of a weakling anathema to me. How people perceived me, as some stealthy badass I suppose, was all that mattered. It shakes me to the core to witness how opening up and speaking and living my truth has not only strengthened and emboldened me somehow, but also reduced the torrent of anxiety I had caused myself for far too long. Weird.

Gone are the days when I'm afraid to admit I don't have all the answers. Gone are the days of not caving into "mom guilt" or that last ice cream sundae cone in the freezer. After reading, Daring Greatly *by Brene Brown, subsequently watching her TedTalk on vulnerability, and currently trudging through the murkiness of a breast cancer diagnoses, I can honestly say I see the light. I'm the most vulnerable I've ever been after half a century on this earth. Because of all of this, instead of resisting the urge to be seen as weak, I've become a person who can embrace, identify, and learn from my vulnerabilities . . . and there are a few!*

So what makes us vulnerable? Brown suggests that our shame and fear of "I'm not _____ enough" denies us the opportunity to embrace vulnerability. The one thing that keeps us from self worth is our fear of disconnectedness. Once we doubt ourselves, we've doomed ourselves to the reality our minds create. The good news is that we have the power to rewrite our realities and shift our mindsets. Identify those "Negative Nelly" thoughts and ask ourselves, "Is this true?" "What makes this true?" And, once we learn that our fears are completely baseless, we can rewrite the fear statements into positive affirmations.

Point blank, having the courage to be imperfect, having the compassion to be kind to ourselves first and then to others, and having the connection as a result of authenticity allows us to be willing to let go of the antiquated beliefs about what we thought we were supposed to be and fully embrace vulnerability. It's not necessarily uncomfortable, it's just necessary.

Becoming willing to say "I love you" first, investing in a relationship that may or may not work out, tiptoeing out on the limb to see how far it bends before it breaks happens when we embrace our "vulnerable" self. What I've learned through life's many adventures is that while vulnerability is at the core of our shame and fear and unworthiness, it is also the birthplace of love, creativity, joy, and belonging.

How do we mesh these counterintuitive beliefs? This has been quite a slugfest for me, but I have come to understand what it means to truly live life wholeheartedly. Warts and all. We can't selectively numb our feelings. When we numb down all the scary emotions of fear, shame, and unworthiness, we also slam the door on golden opportunities for joy, happiness, and gratitude.

Far too often, I've allowed myself to tumble down that rabbit hole of self misery. Then? We become miserable, seeking purpose and meaning, thus plunging headfirst into some crazy cyclone of emotions, and the cycle of struggle continues.

The more afraid we are, the more vulnerable we are. We desperately assign certainty to the uncertain. We want to live vicariously through our kids, free from all of our imperfections. I'll reiterate. This is the most vulnerable I've ever been in my life. Luckily, I'm seasoned with super secret imperfection spices and wired for struggle, but make no mistake—we're all fine. We're all enough. Just the way we are.

Be authentic.

Be real.

Be you.

Love with your whole heart.

Practice gratitude and joy.

Live fearlessly.

Tell yourself endlessly, "I am enough."

Let yourself be seen.

There's not a better model.

Be a warrior.

You've got this.

So, what happens next? The dots need to be connected. It's a chain that can't be broken, as much as I'd like to forget this whole ordeal. We move on. We become better. I'm a big fan of alliteration, and I've come up with some "C" words to combat the cruelty of the big "C" itself:

- Control
- Clarity
- Confidence
- Commitment
- Compassion
- Cured

None of these works in isolation; that's why we play "connect the dots." Connected dots make me happy. Like us, working together in unison to lift one another up, little pixels create a complete and exquisite portrait.

Control

It's the last thing you have when you are fighting cancer. It's the one thing you crave the most. It's especially devastating to a Type A control freak like me. To have one teeny iota of control over what's happening *to* you is what you desire. I'm not talking about the "control freak control" anymore. That's gone. It boils down to the ability to exercise some self-control even though outside forces calling all of the shots. You can't stop nausea from heaving in your stomach. You can't stop the fatigue from squashing you down. You can't control spontaneous bouts of bawling at a McDonald's commercial. This is when the power of meditation and mindfulness saved me. My anxiety attacks in the aftermath of my cancer treatments almost destroyed relationships, derailed some professional choices, and paralyzed me from moving forward. ALMOST. To gain control over my thinking again, and subsequent actions or inactions, I picked up a book recommended to me by a dear and supportive friend, *The Emotional Life of the Brain* by Richard Davidson and Sharon Begley. Through it, I learned that by "tuning in," we can regain power over our thoughts, and our executive functions, like working memory, mental flexibility, and self-control. It taught me the extent to which trauma and adversity can scientifically impact brain function. What I gleaned from the reading was a powerful understanding of the science behind how our brain deals with trauma, adversity, and challenge.

I also embarked, rather clumsily mind you, on mindfulness practices. I started with daybreak and day's end gratitude practices. Before hitting the pillow each night, I recollected three positive things that happened during the day. It could have been anything from someone opening a door for me, a meal shared, laughter, or even a hug. Starting with small gratitudes can lead to bigger and more meaningful gratitudes in days to follow. It quieted my mind and allowed me to fall into much needed, restful sleep. Then, in the morning, before getting out of bed, I laid on my side and quietly prepared my thoughts for a productive day with three things, events, or people for which or whom I was grateful. In bringing those three memories to life, I was able to hone in on the senses. What did I see, hear, smell, taste, feel when I thought about those three things? It literally took only minutes to practice this, but it was critical to rewiring my brain. We get so caught up in our own cancer-related thinking that we bypass opportunities to tune in to moments of connection. A practice so simple but incredibly impactful in regaining control over our minds, our thoughts, and our lives.

Clarity

Journaling: gratitude journals, spiral notebooks, bullet journals, digital—whatever format works best for you and will result in frequent visits and entries, do it! Research shows that writing as an expression of feeling can be therapeutic and cathartic. I love technology; it is an integral component of my everyday life. And while there are innumerable digital resources to record thoughts and memories, there is something to be said about the physical act of putting pen to paper and the healing process. Cleansing and coping. Plus, the colorful markers are fun when you get into a creative doodling groove.

Writing saved my life. Writing became my salvation. Writing replaced my pain medication. Writing provided therapy. No one ever read my writing until now. But I've written all my life. I have reams of handwritten journals sitting at the bottom of an old cedar chest, most of which I've ignored until recently. When you're a teen, when you've been grounded over and over for various infractions, you get bored sitting at home, trying to Humpty Dumpty yourself back together again. I wrote letters to my friends. I wrote blasts to a father who was painfully absent. I wrote sonnets and plays to a love beyond my reach and an entire anthology of poetry—all from the angsty heart of a kid in turmoil. No one has ever read it but me. It mattered to no one but me until now. Going through those old handwritten journals, sometimes filled with prose of teen disquietude, sometimes filled with hope and fantastical teen dreaming, were reflections of the tumultuous waters of my experiences growing up. At any rate, it offered clarity that this cancer thing was not my first rodeo with trauma. I could handle it.

There are a host of scholarly articles and research extolling the benefits of writing on the psyche. Traumatic events, encounters with adversity, or dealing with something like cancer can all be linked to both psychological and additional physical health problems. Writing about adversity is called expressive writing. Writing is not a cure-all. Remember? I said I didn't have any panaceas. No cure-all. That said, I've been writing all my life. It was my drug of choice when something went awry. It seemed simpler to express something through written thought than grab the latest and greatest pharmatucial to help alleviate my angst and suffering. For me and many like me, writing about something weighing heavily on our minds helped foster an intellectual process—the act of constructing a story about a traumatic event—and helped us break free of the endless mental cycling more typical of brooding or rumination. No more dwelling on things. No more anger or guilt. No more sadness or looming clouds. Write it down; return to it if you need to. Find clarity. Truth be told, much like the benefits of exercise on stress reduction, I noticed a negative shift when I stopped writing. Angst brewed. Clarity fogged. Words, often hurtful, flew from my mouth in verbal vomit without considering the ramifications. When I started writing about my experiences, I found it much easier to talk about them with others. Nothing was bottled up because I had already shared things in my journals, my social media posts, my blog, and now my book. My open book.

Like journaling, mindfulness practices serve as another tool in regaining clarity. Learning how the mind works helps with both control and clarity. In my pre-cancer life, when anxiety hit, I found myself fighting it, pushing it down. Eating it. Literally, sometimes. Through mindfulness practice, I now embrace it. Clearly, I'm still a work in progress. That's why they call it *practice*. Breathe deeply through a challenging moment. It might be heart palpitations, tense muscles, irrational thought, or rapid-fire breathing. Deep breath in for the count of five. Own the feeling. Don't run from it; don't hide from it. Brain research illustrates the effects of prolonged trauma and stress on the brain. When it happens and we're experiencing panic or stress, our amygdala, the part of the brain responsible for emotion, survival instincts, and memory, is hijacked. By engaging the prefrontal cortex of our brain, we overcome the amygdala hijack. Breathing through a moment and focusing on each inhale and exhale allows us to let go of the past, bring us back to the present, and immediately kick out negative self-talk. This took me a long time, and much repetition, to master. Now, it's like brushing my teeth. Each morning upon waking, I practice gratitudes. At any time of the day, if a fleeting thought leads me into that dreaded anxiety abyss, I quiet my brain, breathe deeply, engage the moment, and come back to my present state of mind. This takes five to ten minutes tops each time. The beauty of all of this is that science supports mindfulness practice. Long-term meditators are able to recover from negative events much more quickly than non-meditators. Physical parts of our brains can't tell the difference between the physical and imagined stimuli, so it is easier to control with our practices. When we train our minds for greater resilience, we participate in the fundamentals for training a healthy mind. In the time that has passed since completing my treatments, I have been armed with tools necessary for rethinking and kicking anxiety, and subsequent bouts of depression, to the curb. It's returning in tiny increments at a time, but it's the clarity ticket every warrior princess wants to hold.

Confidence

It bears mentioning again: I don't want to be a survivor; I want to be a thriver—kick it all to the curb and be the strongest and most determined version of myself. Repeat after me—"I owe it to myself." You do. You are worthy of self-compassion. It doesn't always seem crystal clear. Confidence can seem beyond reach, especially when mired in trauma. The word "trauma" is a derivative of the Greek word for "wound." There's that attraction to Greek etymology again. This of course encompasses physical, psychological, and emotional ordeals. One commonality between all types of trauma is that it interferes with the daily functioning of a person's life, sometimes to drastic degrees of severity. Again, that voracious, inquisitive mind of mine sought out guidance in my, "Yeah, but how?" questions about how to get my warrior princess back in the driver's seat. Turns out, taking these steps can help us regain our confidence when we're attempting to keep one nostril above water to eventually wield that sword and shield again.

1. Repeat after me: "My past does not define me."
2. Embrace healing beliefs to replace negative self-talk.
3. Slow and steady wins the race. Baby steps. Always forward.
4. Forgive freely—yourself and others.
5. Take time for self-care and practice self-love.

6. Keep close, positive circles of people who uplift you and encourage healing.
7. Trust life again and the people and experiences that accompany it. Life is best when served lived and lived well!
8. Liberate yourself through acceptance of your personal adversity; suffering is a normal, yet uncomfortable, component of living.

It goes without saying that some of these steps are easier than others, depending on our situations. It takes a concerted effort. We may stumble. We may fall. My question to you is, "Are you worth it?" My unequivocal answer? "Absolutely, yes!"

Confidence blossoms from turning negatives into positives: taking cancer, something that could and does kill, and turning it into a life force; taking hatred and turning it into love and forgiveness; taking ignorance and turning it into respect. In true warrior fashion, sometimes you just need to stick your nose to the ground and GO. Just GO. You almost need blinders on at times but not blinders that keep you from seeing everything beautiful that surrounds you. Embrace those who drive your horizons wider, broader, and more plentiful. Seek understanding what others need when trudging through adversity; how can we reach out to them? That's when confidence seeps through the cracks in our souls.

Ah, Maya Angelou, you never fail to provide the wisest words that perfectly sum up what I want to say.

"My mission in life is not to merely survive, but to thrive; and to do so with passion, some compassion, some humor, and some style."

Commitment

Much like before all of this went down, I had seemingly infinite commitments: family, job, relationships, health, volunteerism, financial, love. We all do this. When you're jolted into outer space for a little galactic puke fest, the only commitment you can make is to try to keep your lunch down, try to remember to change your underwear each day, or try to smile when every joint in your body aches. And often, in isolation. One step at a time.

When you reach the other side of the tunnel and you can actually see the light, smell the flowers, and feel the breeze on your face, that's the point when you can start making commitments again. Commitments to thriving and a real life, not just to surviving the mucky muck. It takes time. I'll be the first to admit, I was not patient with myself in this process. I wanted to be done-zo with all the mucky muck and get back to actually caring about my undies and getting this mid-life bod back into action again.

Having spent most of my professional life in the world of education, I had a great deal of background knowledge in setting goals, with colleagues, as a system, and with students alike. So, I reached into my skill set closet for something I already knew: S.M.A.R.T. goals. I would assume that anyone dealing with strategic planning in business or education, or anyone working with clients in health care or fitness/wellness programs, has heard about these. You can Google them. They are goals that, in theory, offer accountability and reality to the jumbled to-do lists percolating in your brain. S.M.A.R.T. stands for *Specific, Measurable, Attainable, Realistic/Relevant,* and *Time-bound.*

Specific—Goals should be written in simple language and clearly define what you are going to do. When goals are too broad (e.g. I want to lose weight, become rich, be famous), they lack focus, and it is tough to attach action steps to them.

Measurable—Goals should be measurable so that you have tangible evidence that you have accomplished the goal. There are usually several short-term or smaller measurements built into the goal. Celebrating small successes keep us focused on the larger prize.

Attainable—Goals should be achievable; they should stretch you slightly so you feel challenged but defined well enough so that you can achieve them. It helps to possess the appropriate knowledge, skills, and capabilities necessary to achieve the goal.

Realistic/Relevant—Goals should be reasonable and meaningful. If goals are arbitrary or unlikely (so much for becoming a world class ballerina), they are likely to be pushed aside and forgotten.

Time-bound—Goals should be linked to a time frame that creates a practical sense of urgency or results in necessary tension between the current reality and the vision of the goal that results in action being taken. Without such tension, the goal is unlikely to produce an outcome pertinent to the goal.

Furthermore, I would suggest taking those goals a couple of steps further; make them S.M.A.R.T.E.R.:

Evaluative—Evaluate the goal if the action steps seem to go around and around without getting anywhere. They're obviously not helping to reach your goals; they're just making you dizzy.

Revisable—Once goals are evaluated (Were they too big? Too unmotivating? Too daunting? Too out there?), they can be revised.

Making small shifts in action steps can assist in getting back on track. Then, when ready, shoot for the moon with the original goal.

Case in point: A year after my diagnosis, six months following chemo, and about two months after completing radiation, we were celebrating New Year's. I, like millions of people, sketched out those adorable little New Year's Resolutions. My S.M.A.R.T.E.R. goal was to drop fifty pounds by the following new year, which gave me a year to accomplish the goal (time-bound, realistic, specific). How would I attain and measure this goal? I joined a weight loss competition at the local gym. Eight weeks. Weekly weigh-ins. Pants that actually fit sans the muffin top. I had weekly workouts planned. I carefully crafted healthy meals at home and during road trips for work. I failed miserably. Here's where *evaluative* and *revisable* come into play. You know how you walk into the grocery store with the best of intentions to purchase only what's on the list? And then you walk out with a cart full of absolutely must-have deals? You completely underestimated the power and appeal of the sales, right? Well, that was me, only I completely underestimated the power and longevity of fatigue and overall lapse in physical strength, borderline depression, and chaotic thinking. I evaluated and revised. I've given myself permission, practiced a little compassion for my healing, and rebooted my goal, but I shifted the action plan around a bit. More gentle yoga and increased walking to start. Make it through a whole day at work and have the ability to stay awake past eight o'clock and maintain a decent night's sleep without all of the anxiety aerobics that frequently took place. Gradually cut out comfort foods and slam those healthy greens. (Kale and I are still warming up to each other.) This is where I find myself. A work in progress, and progress is good. More energy each day, more strength in muscles, less fatigue, and who knew TV could actually be enjoyable after 8:00? Just an example of how we don't need to throw the baby out with the bath water and chuck the whole plan when we stumble. Get back up, dust yourself off, and carry on.

Setting goals is great. What can I do to keep myself in check? I circle back to journaling. Daily logs help monitor progress. Write it down. They also help us see time frames or triggers that challenge our advancement so we can deal with them effectively and proactively. Journaling helps strengthen our intentions. They are progress monitoring aids in learning and practicing moderation, acquiring and recording new information, and thinking for the long haul. The magic happens outside of our comfort zones. Well, cancer pushes you about as far out of your comfort zone and into the stratosphere as you can possibly get. Through this process, though, I would argue that when we regain that power, we can redefine our comfort zones. On our own terms. And then stretch beyond them toward even more growth. I set goals, monitored my progress, and celebrated every little success along the way. Yay for new pants that fit! I'm clearly not all the way there yet, but hey! We're all works in progress, right? Remember that.

Compassion

I'll admit it. I was a real ballbuster. Ask anyone who knows me. Sometimes a wolf. Sometimes a pitbull. I can be kind and docile, and the minute I get riled up, or I get pinned against the wall, I can pounce. I admit, somewhat shamefully, that it was hard to show compassion, especially toward people I didn't understand, and I didn't see the potential for my growth in these situations. Instead, I felt threatened. I lacked compassion . . . and compromise. Not so much anymore. By no means was this transformation a solo effort. I never thought I needed help, but I was irrefutably wrong. I relied heavily on professionals, trusted experts, and close friends and family to gain invaluable insights to make a change. I can't count the number of individuals who reached out and showed me countless acts of compassion (even if I didn't particularly deserve it). Compassion is some compelling and humbling stuff. At the same time I was listening first to understand, by practicing compassion for others and self, I learned to understand myself more deeply. They killed the old me with kindness, and for that I am forever grateful. Connections were transformed into an unintended sisterhood. Connections were strengthened for secure and tighter circles of friends and family. Pretty commanding weapons for the greater good, I would argue.

The thing about living a life with cancer is that it connects you to people you never thought it would. I remember being pregnant with each of my kids, and suddenly a trip to the grocery store or mall became a gallery walk of pregnant women. I had never noticed all of the baby bumps until I had one (and it was more like a small condo than a cute little baby bump, by the way). The same applies to cancer. You notice the bald heads, you notice the absent eyebrows and lashes, and you notice the asymmetry in upper bodies post-op. It's weird. I firmly believe this awareness builds compassion. It also builds connection. I recently learned about a colleague who was about to embark on her own journey. Funny how that happens. I immediately leaped into support net mode—offering ears, shoulders, and arms for hugs of comfort, my personal email, and limiting the amount of information and advice. . . until requested. She sent me this email:

Kaye,

Again, thank you for taking some time with me the other day. It felt surprisingly good to come in . . . Maybe not top of my game, but I will get there.

The interesting thing I noticed when I got home was that I felt different somehow. I couldn't quite put my finger on it, but then I realized what it was. Hope . . . a very small flicker and still very distant, but it had not been there in any way until after I talked with you. And that hope was not about the outcome of the cancer. It was that one day, I won't feel like this anymore. That I will get to the other side of this. Anyway, that's because of you. So, that's what I am thanking you for.

Side note: I then went outside to sit and enjoy some peace for a bit, and out of the blue, a dragonfly came and put on a show for me . . . spinning and flying and dipping. I am a believer in the universe and that we are all connected and that these sort of gifts are there for us.

This from the interweb: The dragonfly, in almost every part of the world, symbolizes change and change in the perspective of self realization. The kind of change that has its source in mental and emotional maturity and the understanding of the deeper meaning of life.

I love that! BTW, the podcast was really good and timely. Thank you!

This is something I can't reiterate enough: you do not have to walk alone. There are multitudes of people willing to help. It takes a quick gulp in the throat and headstrong warrior determination to ask. It takes a huge dose of warrior princess bravery to ask for help. Again, in coming to terms with my own grief, I now seek to help others trudging through their own challenges. That is why fellow thriver sisters and I, dissatisfied with gaps in regional cancer emotional advocacy, are convening to create some type of regional ad hoc support group, something like a *Surviving to Thriving* service. Rightfully so, I had thought about a warrior princess-themed service, but (1) it's already taken, and (2) we want to assist ALL (men and women) going through the perils of a cancer battle. The goal is to address the elephant in the room, the stuff no one talks about once you're through the proverbial woods, and to uplift one another in a judgement-free zone, like Planet Fitness without all the sweaty smelliness. The aftermath . . . the *so what, now what?* phase.

Patience, Grasshopper . . . Google *Karate Kid*. Classic.

Cured

Let me be crystal clear: I may have had cancer, but it will *never* have me. It will not define me. It's part of my DNA now, but it isn't *all* of me. I'm one of the fortunate ones. After that whole battery of tests following treatment and a few minor procedures, I actually have a better handle on what's going on inside my body than most. That's pretty darn lucky. The worst thing I need to deal with now is remembering my pill each day. That's lucky. Physically, my outer appearance is relatively symmetrical, unless there's some uncanny shift in gravity, which I've noticed only occasionally. It's hard to detect that anything drastic happened . . . except that I'm a little less top-heavy than I was . . . and a little perkier. That's lucky. Not everyone has the chance to laugh at themselves and give their prosthetics names, like Foob 1 and Foob 2, for example. Or, so I've heard.

When I was a child, we bellied up on the shag carpet in front of our brand new color TV set and watched one of our favorite shows of the '70s, *Little House on the Prairie.* It was on one of the whopping three channel options we had. Sometimes less is more! The portrayal of a father who lovingly provided for his family was a beautiful little fantasy for me. Seeing sisters who got along pretty well and went through challenges and arguments and "huffing off" tantrums with one another was nice, too. The whole frolicking in the prairie with no concern for wildlife that could readily devour them or that nasty Nellie Olson who made Laura's life routinely miserable was real for me. I connected to that. It was normal.

Fast forward some forty years later, I am taken back to one episode in particular. It was a funeral scene for one of the Ingalls' neighbors, Julia Sanderson (seriously, I had to Google everything but the quote). I do remember that as a child, I was in awe of the great film star, Patricia Neal. She always seemed to portray the most realistic characters. For some reason, I found connection to those characters as I grew up. It was a message that her character,

Julia, had written before she died and was read at her funeral, and for whatever reason, I jotted it down on a napkin we likely got with our pizza for dinner and stuck it away in a little wooden "treasure box" I made in seventh grade Industrial Arts class. Who knew I'd be thinking about my own mortality at age fifty?

It read:

"Remember me with smiles and laughter, for that is how I'll remember you all.
If you can only remember me with tears, then don't remember me at all."

I think about this quote more often than I probably should, but it's the truth. I want people to celebrate me when I'm gone. I want them to smile, reminisce, and laugh recalling some of the ridiculous shenanigans I had gotten myself into. I want them to remember my passion for all of my students. I want them to remember my transformation. I want them to remember my thirst for knowledge. I want them to remember me as a "mother bear"/ helicopter mom. I want them to recall moments when I really ticked them off or challenged their thinking in some way. I want them to hear me audaciously belting out Pat Benatar at the top of my lungs on any given karaoke night. I want them to eat and drink and laugh and dance until they all fall down. Tears can wait.

Fortunately, I have some time to set all of those plans aside. I remember one of the last monthly visits to the doctor. No tests this time. No blood work. Just a routine check up to ensure all was going as planned. No need for pokes and prods. I was able to take the stairs this time with no worries about losing wind or consciousness. As I waited for the notification vibration on my appointment pager to go off, I looked around the chemo wing waiting area. Funny how the stark white walls never phased me when I was sitting there, waiting for my turn to get poisoned or poked. Funny I never noticed the hospital's attempt to provide uplifting, light, soothing music, and vibrant hues in the artwork near the doors entering the treatment rooms. I saw women in caps and scarves and bald heads. Some conversing, most in quiet contemplation. I saw men in wheelchairs, curled over in pain, likely sleeping because of fatigue or the sheer exhaustion of fighting so hard. I saw a young child. Great. Waterworks. That's when the unfairness of all of this hits. Not the kids! No child should *ever* suffer through cancer. EVER. These people were me. I was them. I sat where they now sit. I wondered what was going through their heads. Despair? Hope? Wonder? Relief? Worry about finances? Worry about side effects? Worry about who will pick them up? Worry about making it to the next Christmas? Then, thanks to the pager/buzzer thing, I snapped back to my side of the waiting area—the more hopeful, follow-up section of the oncology floor.

Once again, I was ready for my allotted one thousand questions. It happened almost every appointment. I kept my list on my phone. This time was different, though. This time, there was no list on my phone. This time, there was more hope than worry. There was more strength than fatigue. For some reason, the sun shined a little brighter for this appointment than in the past. My oncologist entered the room in his typical, avuncular manner. After our ceremonial welcoming handshake and some small talk about how

I was feeling, he rummaged through my medical records on the computer for the hundredth time. We spoke briefly about how my medication was treating me, how my neuropathy was progressing, how my fatigue was improving, and then he asked the question he always seemed reticent to ask in the past: "Everything is looking good. Any questions for me?" I could almost see him cringe, bracing himself as if to say, "Okay. Hit me. I know the question typhoon is coming."

"So . . . am I *cured*?"

Crap. I could feel the tears well up in my eyes. It was really the only question I had at the moment. It was the only one remaining that I truly needed an answer to. He reached out and put his hand on my shoulder and tenderly smiled. "How old are you now? Fifty-one? I'll let you know in forty-nine more years."

Dear Kaye and Dave,

Just a note to cheer you on and let you know you're in our thoughts and prayers as you take on this challenge. Along with your fabulous, loving husband and family, we've got your back.

My sister battled breast cancer at the age of fifty, too. After a mastectomy with axillary lymph node dissection with several positive nodes as well as reconstructive surgery and chemo, she is now, at age sixty-six, healthier than she has ever been. She was up for the challenge, and so are you! You've got this, girl!

Please don't hesitate to call on us if you need anything. I know everybody says this, but I mean every word of it.

Even though ice fishing is over for the season (sniff, sniff), we will have plenty of time this summer to chill at the lake. I'm looking forward to it with every passing day.

You take care of yourself, and let Dave wait on you hand and foot (*smiles). He's such a great guy. I'm sure he's the most caring and compassionate nurse you'll ever have!

Best wishes,

J & G

Final Thoughts: The Battle is Never Done

Sometimes life knocks you on your ass . . . get up, get up, get up!
Happiness is not the absence of problems,
it's the ability to deal with them.
~Steven Maraboli~

Warrior princesses. We fight. We're flawed. Sometimes we sport some glorious and gnarly tattoos. Amazons were big on tattoos. There were a lot of them—beautifully, lovingly detailed tattoos in the images of Scythian women (Amazon warrior princesses) on vase paintings. Ancient Greek historians described the tattooing practices of the culturally related tribes of Ephesus, home of the Amazons. They could have been initiations, they could have been just for decoration, they could have represented special experiences, either in reality or dreams. No one really knows; it's mythology, afterall. All we can assume is that they were heavily tattooed, mostly with real and fantastical animals and geometric designs. Tattoos tell a story. Granted, they're not for everyone. I have several, all chosen after the age of thirty . . . probably because I was too busy raising kids to make any appointments at my local tattoo shop. Johnny Depp, heavily tattooed, once said, "My skin is my journal, and the tattoos are the stories."

A year after my diagnosis and subsequent treatment, I entered a contest to connect with a regional tattoo artist who donated their time and talents to the P.Ink Day initiative. This incredible opportunity affords a limited number of women an all-expenses paid mastectomy tattoo . . . a unique way to tell the story of their battle, the story of their triumph over a vicious, relentless enemy. Truthfully, I never expected to be selected. Six months later, I learned I was chosen, and in fall of 2018—a full year and some change of hellish whiplash, I'll enter a new adventure of storytelling. And, let me tell you, it's going to be a doozy. Paired with a talented artist, I will have yet one more way to tell my story. It will become one of the rays of light to shine through all of this darkness.

Bottom line, regardless of princess moniker, we warriors are fierce. By surviving the battle of adversity, be it cancer or bankruptcy or mental health challenges or any other personal chaos, we've all earned our armor. Kinks and dents. Scars and burns. We've multiplied our allies. We've learned how to jump back up after being flung off our steeds by our enemies' swords. And continue the battle. We've broadened our skills to transition from surviving to thriving. And, we've earned the right to do what we want. Battle on, warriors, battle on.

Bibliography

Brown, Brené. *Daring Greatly: How the Courage to Be Vulnerable Transforms the Way We Live, Love, Parent, and Lead.* New York: Avery, 2012.

Covey, Stephen R. *The 7 Habits of Highly Effective People: Restoring the Character Ethic.* [Rev. ed.]. New York: Free Press, 2004.

Davidson, Richard J., and Sharon Begley. 2012. *The Emotional Life of Your Brain: How its Unique Patterns Affect the Way You Think, Feel, and Live--and How You Can Change Them.* New York: Hudson Street Press.

Estés, Clarissa Pinkola. *Women Who Run with the Wolves: Myths and Stories of the Wild Woman Archetype.* New York: Ballantine Books, 1992.

Mayor, Adrienne. *The Amazons: Lives and Legends of Warrior Women across the Ancient World.* Princeton: Princeton University Press, 2016.

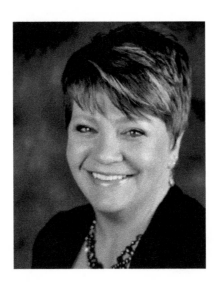

KAYE HENRICKSON is a wife, mother, sister, daughter, friend. And oh, a breast cancer survivor. Check that, she's a warrior princess thriver. Kaye has served in the education field her entire career, sharing her passion for writing, learning, and creative expression with learners of all ages. Kaye shares her story with audiences, both large and small, with hopes of helping people unleash their own inner warrior, regardless of the adversity they face. Kaye spends her time away from the written word with her best friend, Dave, family and friends, and of course, their rescue princess pooch, Geneva. Preferably, somewhere near woods or water.